Feeling Tired All the Time

Co

Feeling Tired All the Time

COMPLETELY REVISED AND UPDATED

Dr Joe Fitzgibbon

Newleaf

Published by

Newleaf

an imprint of

Gill & Macmillan Ltd

Hume Avenue, Park West, Dublin 12

with associated companies throughout the world

www.gillmacmillan.ie

© Dr Joe Fitzgibbon 1993, 2001

0 7171 3285 4

Print origination by O'K Graphic Design, Dublin

Printed by ColourBooks Ltd, Dublin

This book is typeset in 10/12.5 pt Garamond Book

The paper used in this book comes from the wood pulp of managed forests. For every tree felled, at least one tree is planted, thereby renewing natural resources.

A CIP catalogue record for this book is available from the British Library.

6 8 10 9 7

Contents

Preface

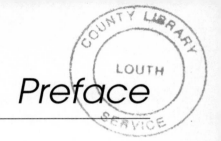

One of my teachers passed a rather casual remark when I was a medical student. It stuck with me. He said that 50 per cent of medical knowledge becomes obsolete after five years! He was referring, of course, to the fact that the practice of medicine is in a state of constant evolution, with new advances being made all the time. This may seem like a rather obvious statement to make, but the truth of it is clearly brought home to me as I look back on the first edition of *Feeling Tired All the Time*: it's starting to look obsolete! So much has changed since it first appeared some eight years ago, particularly in relation to chronic fatigue syndrome (CFS). For example, the Centre for Disease Control (USA) revised the definition of CFS in 1994, and the Royal Colleges of Physicians, Psychiatrists and General Practitioners (UK) published a joint landmark report on CFS in 1996. Then, in 1999, the Irish College of General Practitioners included a module on CFS in their new diploma in therapeutics. Meanwhile, over 700 articles dealing with CFS have appeared in the medical literature; and I have had the benefit of another eight years of clinical experience with fatigued patients. The time has come to put pen to paper again.

Feedback from the first edition was very encouraging. Many said they enjoyed the simple and concise style of writing. They also found the material easy to understand. This second edition contains much by way of new information. New sections have been added, and many others have been expanded. However, every effort has been made to keep the information simple and accessible. I hope you will find it so.

Introduction

'Doctor, I feel tired all the time' is the single most common complaint presented by patients to their doctors. This has been confirmed by studies in the UK and the USA, in which up to 20 per cent of men and 30 per cent of women identified themselves as having the complaint. We all experience fatigue as a transient phenomenon, particularly during times of physical and emotional stress, and most of us recover full strength, without help, once the affliction has passed. But when fatigue becomes chronic — to wake in the morning feeling as if you haven't slept all night, barely able to pull your body out of bed, and having to drag yourself through the day, trying as best you can to perform your basic duties — it can be a distressing and debilitating symptom. A normal social life is out of the question.

However, you've been to your doctor, but with nothing to show for your symptoms, apart from a story which is difficult to communicate, let alone understand. All the tests are normal and you've been told, 'There's nothing wrong. Perhaps it's all in your head!' But where do you go from here? 'Try harder', they say, supposing that all you need is more motivation. The prod is hurtful. Nevertheless, you try harder, but you still cannot find the elusive energy, which is by now only a distant memory. In fact, trying harder makes you feel worse.

Some manage to carry on for years, being careful to hide their true state from those around them. Others simply cannot put themselves through any more. They feel totally drained. Even the most basic personal and domestic tasks seem too much. A few withdraw completely, becoming house-bound, or even bed-bound. Relationships become strained as family and friends strive to understand what they cannot see. In fact, they often think you look just fine. Many who have suffered like this will say that they have lost valuable years; some have lost their jobs, others their marriages; and some, in the pits of despair, have taken their own lives.

The difficulty facing doctors was well summarised in a *British*

Introduction

Medical Journal editorial: 'There is no clinical problem more demanding of the art of medicine than the management of lassitude (fatigue).' This is so because it is a subjective symptom. It cannot be demonstrated objectively by either physical examination or laboratory tests. It gives the doctor nothing to go on but your word. If you are taken seriously, a long list of possible diagnoses must be considered — from the apparently trivial, to the more ominous life-threatening diseases.

Stress and depression are reported to be the most common causes of fatigue. For this reason, they will figure prominently in any balanced discussion on the subject. But fatigue has many other explanations, some of which, in spite of being easy to investigate and simple to treat, are seldom considered. Another problem is that some doctors still deny the existence of a chronic fatigue syndrome. Perhaps this explains, at least in part, why patients with fatigue are so quickly and unreasonably dismissed as being depressed or stressed. The brunt of this common practice has been borne by the most severely affected patients. 'Of course I'm depressed', they argue in frustration, 'it's because I feel so tired all the time.' But the cold shoulder remains and the patient turns in desperation to anyone who offers even a glimmer of hope. They are exceedingly vulnerable now and many have spent small fortunes in their quest for relief.

This book is an introduction to the common and treatable causes of fatigue. It hopes to provide you with a clear understanding of just why it is you feel so tired, and suggests means by which you can help yourself back towards a normal, healthy and energetic life.

Section 1

Putting Fatigue in Context

1 The Complex Problem of Fatigue

It would be helpful, as we start out, to define what we mean by fatigue and to give it some context. Fatigue is a symptom, a subjective feeling. We say 'I *feel* tired.' Nobody else can see our tiredness; we have to tell them what it feels like. Similarly, when we feel pain or feel nauseous or feel dizzy, we are feeling things that others cannot see. Signs of disease, on the other hand, are the physical manifestations of illness. They are more objective, and other people can see them, especially those with a trained eye. Indeed, sometimes the patient cannot see the sign, they only feel the symptoms.

Jaundice, for example, is a definite sign of disease. It usually means there is something wrong with your liver. You can see the yellow in the eyes where there should be white. Similarly, the rash of meningitis, the swollen tonsils of a streptococcal throat, and the red streaming eyes of an allergic reaction are all signs that other people can see and which help doctors to make a diagnosis. Unfortunately, there are no signs of fatigue, only a dreadful feeling. This is the first reason why it can be such a difficult problem to diagnose.

When doctors are formulating a diagnosis, they take a detailed account of your symptoms (your feelings). Then they examine you for physical signs, and then, if need be, they order tests. These medical tests are simply another attempt to obtain objective evidence of disease. Thus a high blood sugar would suggest diabetes, and a kidney stone on X-ray would explain renal colic. Unfortunately, there are no laboratory tests that can diagnose or measure fatigue; and, in the vast majority of cases, all the investigations are normal. This is the second reason why fatigue is so difficult to diagnose. The third reason is this: fatigue may accompany virtually any disease state. It is truly a non-specific symptom.

Fatigue, therefore, is a subjective symptom that shows no signs of disease: it cannot be measured or confirmed by investigation, and it may be part and parcel of any disease you care to think of. To quote again from a *British Medical Journal* editorial, this is why the doctor's reaction to the fatigued patient 'is frequently one of frustration and helplessness, since they know the bewildering variety of causes, the many psychological factors, and the frequent impotence of medical treatment'.

I believe that the 'impotence of medical treatment' is not quite as bad as it used to be, but some of the old attitudes remain. In their frustration and helplessness, some doctors have fallen into a scientific trap, a professional comfort zone, so to speak. This is an arrogant and dark place where otherwise brilliant minds become unstuck through the limitations of their machines. If they cannot measure it objectively in the laboratory, they are inclined to dismiss it. This is why you might be told, 'There is nothing wrong with you.' What you should be told, of course, is: 'Our technology has not yet reached the point where we can explain your symptoms.'

OK, so let us now take a look at your fatigue. And let us start by putting it into some sort of perspective. To help us with this task, I suggest we conduct a hypothetical survey of an entire community. You will see that you are not alone in your fatigue.

Fatigue — a hypothetical community survey

For argument's sake, we will study a small town with a population of, say, 2,000 people, and we will ask each member of this community to fill out a health questionnaire. The first and obvious finding would be this: they would all know what it's like to feel tired. After all, they would say fatigue is a universal experience. But we are not interested in this 'normal tiredness'. We are more concerned with those who feel tired *all* or *most* of the time, and whose quality of life is significantly impaired as a result. One-fifth of the men and one-third of the women in this survey would admit to this sort of tiredness. In other words, some 500 of these 2,000 people would be feeling tired at any one point in time.

Sadly, only one in five of these will go to a doctor for help. The others will struggle on as best they can.

It is likely that those who stay away from doctors do so because they are afraid their tiredness would be construed as trivial and that they would be quickly dismissed. Others may fear being told that their symptoms are 'all in your mind'. Finally, others may avoid going to the doctor in the belief that nothing can be done to help. It must be said, to our shame, that these fears and attitudes originated first in doctors, and that patients only learned of them afterwards through bitter experience. In any case, only 100 of our original 500 fatigued people will end up with the doctor. It is important to remember that these patients present with a chief complaint of feeling tired all the time, in other words, this is the primary reason they are going to see the doctor. You will see the relevance of this shortly.

Fatigue — 100 hypothetical patients

Let us now follow these patients and see what happens to them. What sort of diagnoses do they end up with? Let us also ensure that they are given the benefit of the very best medical evaluation. As alluded to above, this would include a detailed clinical history, followed by a physical examination and appropriate laboratory tests. They would also have an examination of their mental state to elicit any features of psychological distress. Finally, if necessary, the patient would be referred to a specialist for a second opinion.

Would you be surprised to learn that up to 70 per cent of our patients will be given an accurate psychiatric diagnosis? Depression is the most common disorder identified in those who present with fatigue. This is followed closely by anxiety, panic and phobic disorders. A much smaller percentage is found to have somatisation (hysteria) or some other psychiatric disorder. These are specific and positive diagnoses; they are made on the basis of firm evidence of psychiatric symptomatology, and many patients respond well to appropriate treatment. The outlook is excellent for most of them.

Reassuringly, less than 5 per cent of our patients will be given a physical diagnosis, such as a low blood count, an underactive thyroid, or worse. That leaves us with a full 25 per cent who cannot be classified into physical or psychiatric categories. Thus, we have what one researcher has called an 'irreducible minority' of patients whose fatigue cannot be explained by physician or psychiatrist. This is what we mean when we speak of chronic unexplained fatigue.

Five patients from this group could turn out to have a chronic fatigue syndrome; a similar number will have fibromyalgia (a related disorder); and the remainder will end up with the rather unsatisfactory label of idiopathic (we-don't-know-the-cause-of-it) fatigue. There is no contradiction in saying that some patients with unexplained fatigue have chronic fatigue syndrome or fibromyalgia, for we are still unable to explain these conditions. Nevertheless, the diagnostic labels are useful in that they allow us to recognise patients who have a specific cluster of symptoms and offer them some practical help towards recovery.

The results of our survey are summarised in Table 1. You will see that they give this book its basic structure. We will deal with each category in turn, starting with the psychological and psychiatric explanations of fatigue in Section 2(i) and the physical explanations in Section 2(ii). In Section 4 we will deal with chronic debilitating fatigue of unknown origin. But before we do that we will examine the treatable causes of fatigue that are frequently overlooked in the assessment of the fatigued patient. These appear in Section 3 under the general headings of sleep, diet, germs and chemicals. These explanations of fatigue do not appear in our survey because the researchers didn't ask about them! Perhaps these forgotten causes were hidden among those who were said to have idiopathic fatigue. We must remember, therefore, that fatigue can only remain idiopathic after *all* the other possibilities have been explored. We won't find an explanation for your tiredness if we don't look for one!

Do not accept the label of idiopathic fatigue until you are sure that all other possibilities have been considered.

Fatigue — one real life case history

So much for population studies, but how should we approach *your* specific case? We are faced with so many possible explanations. Well, as always in medicine, we start with the clinical history. Have a read through the following example. In many ways it is quite typical and, as you would expect, in some ways it is unique.

Table 1.

Population of 2,000	• All will have experienced transient fatigue.
Of these 2,000	• 500 will complain of significant fatigue all or most of the time.
Of these 500	• 400 will struggle on as best they can and avoid doctors. 100 will seek medical help.
Of these 100	• 70 will have a psychiatric diagnosis and do well with treatment. • 5 will have a physical condition, such as anaemia. • 25 will have a fatigue that defies explanation.
Of the 70 with psychiatric diagnoses	• 40 will have depression. • 25 will have anxiety, panic or a phobic condition. • 5 will have hysteria or a related disorder.
Of the 25 with unexplained fatigue	• 1-5 will have a chronic fatigue syndrome. • 1-5 will have fibromyalgia. • The remainder will have idiopathic fatigue.

Case history

Allison is a 20-year-old university student living away from home. Attractive, intelligent and well spoken, you would think she has everything going for her. Although her appearance belies the fact, she is actually quite unwell. She complains of feeling tired all the time, and is especially prone to exhaustion following exercise. Even tasks we all take so much for granted, like climbing the stairs or taking lecture notes, have become difficult.

Her problem started, out of the blue, some four years ago. One morning, returning from her daily swim, she felt exceptionally tired. After a few days it was clear that she was not improving, so she went to see her doctor who, finding nothing wrong, arranged her admission to hospital. All sorts of tests were carried out, but with the exception of one ambiguous result, which half-raised the possibility of a viral infection, they drew a blank. She was then sent to a psychiatrist who prescribed an antidepressant, but she stopped taking it because of intolerable side effects. Allison missed a full year of school, but when she did eventually return to her studies, she achieved good enough grades to secure a place in the science faculty at the university.

Although she has some relatively good days, Allison has never really recovered full strength. She is doing her best to complete the current academic year, but her memory and concentration are now affected. She is troubled with forgetfulness and describes herself as being 'muddled' in thought. Recently her fatigue has become more severe, causing her to miss a number of lectures. She is already older than her present classmates, and it's beginning to look as if she might have to drop behind again.

She is, not surprisingly, depressed and weepy. When questioned further, she admits to a host of other symptoms: palpitations, premenstrual tension, painful periods, irritable bowel syndrome, muscle pains, mouth ulcers, indigestion, frequent sore throats and frequent colds. She also describes recurring episodes of feeling 'faint and shivery'; these bouts are relieved temporarily by eating a bar of chocolate or some other sugar-laden food (to which she will readily confess addiction). She supplements this rather inadequate diet with two pints of milk every day and ten mugs of coffee. Her appetite is good and her weight stable, she does not smoke cigarettes or drink alcohol, and she has never taken illegal drugs.

She used to be a lively sort, enjoying the normal activities of teenage years, but that's all changed now. She used to have a boyfriend, but he's gone. He grew impatient. She feels guilty for being ill, for not being able to pull herself out of this dreadful pit, and she's fed up with living at the receiving end of charity. Her family is anxious. They wonder what on earth is going on, and whether there will ever be an end to this nightmare. Allison and those who love her have suffered a great deal. They are not alone in their plight. Neither are you.

No doubt you will have recognised some of your own symptoms here. As you read through the analysis that follows, you will start to pick up some of the clues that could explain your own fatigue.

The analysis

Apart from some details that have been changed to protect her identity, this is sadly a true story. It may seem at first glance to be a hopeless case, but it is not. If we take a closer look at the details of her history, we will find a number of possible explanations for her fatigue, some of which, it must be said, do not appear to have been considered at all. In so doing, we may be able to offer her — for the first time ever — some real hope of a cure.

To start our search we should go back to the beginning, to the days and weeks before her symptoms first appeared. It turns out that she was under considerable stress at the time. She was preparing for an important examination that would determine her future career. She may have felt subject to undue pressure, from home or from within, to succeed academically. When she first came to see me, she was again facing exams — it would not be wise to dismiss this as mere coincidence. Stress of this sort can quickly lead to outright depression, and one of the main complaints of those who are depressed is a feeling of chronic fatigue. The psychiatrist who saw her initially thought that she was depressed. Perhaps she was, and perhaps she still is. She does cry a lot, her sleep pattern is disturbed, and she never did finish her course of antidepressants; but — and this is a very big 'but' — is her depression the cause of her symptoms, or the result of them?

On the other hand, it could be that all her trouble stems from a disturbed sleep pattern *per se*. We know that sleep deprivation has a profound effect on body and brain, and that it will inevitably induce fatigue. She does go to bed a bit on the late side, and it is a long time since she regularly enjoyed wholesome, restorative sleep.

The next thing we should look at is the possibility of a viral infection. You will remember that this prospect was raised early on in the course of her illness. Sometimes a virus can hide itself inside muscle (and other) cells and remain there undetected by both immune system, and laboratory tests for years. Similarly, some viruses disrupt cell function before they are beaten by the immune system, and this disruption can persist long after the virus has been cleared. This could explain her fatigue, muscle pains, exhaustion after exercise, recurrent sore throats and colds.

Her bouts of feeling 'faint and shivery' raise yet another possibility, that of reactive hypoglycaemia (low blood sugar). The clue here is that she craves sweet things. These give her a dramatic rise in blood sugar levels, and although she gets an energy boost from them, it lasts only a short time. When the blood sugar subsequently falls again, it does so precipitously, bringing on faintness, shivering and fatigue. The excessive caffeine she drinks serves only to aggravate the sugar swings, and may be contributing to fatigue in its own right.

Her great preference for milk may also be significant. Patients with food intolerance can become strangely fond of their culprit foods. The chances of fatigue being 'allergic' in origin are greatly increased when other possible symptoms of food intolerance are present. Irritable bowel symptoms, mouth ulcers and indigestion may each be induced by adverse reactions to food. Besides all this, her diet is nutritionally inadequate. It does not supply her with the essential vitamins and minerals that are required for optimal health and energy. Finally — and this is an apprehension frequently voiced by those who have unresolved symptoms — it is possible that some serious disease has been overlooked by her doctor, or is not yet fully manifest.

In any case, whatever the original cause of her fatigue, she now has to cope with additional factors that are bound to have a compounding effect. A recent move away from home, a broken romance, the pressure of exams, the loss of a social life, or wondering whether she can cope with the future, will only worsen her fatigue.

As you can see, fatigue can be a complex dilemma. It is a difficult symptom to live with. It mars the enjoyment of life, interferes with performance, strains relationships, hinders potential and frustrates ambition. To get to its root, in this or in any other case, will require a committed and painstaking effort. This will involve looking at the problem, not just from one angle but from many, taking every possible influence into consideration. If it is going to yield at all, it will yield to patient enquiry.

2   *Normal Energy Levels*

Before we delve any further into the various causes of fatigue, we should take a brief look at so called 'normal' energy levels. In our introductory survey we found that 1,500 people from a community of 2,000 described themselves as *not* feeling tired all the time. Presumably then these 75 per cent of the population are a relatively fit and healthy lot. But how well do they really feel? Let's find out. We can ask them to rate their energy levels for us. For this purpose we will give each one of them a simple visual analogue scale. It looks something like this:

1 | 2 | 3 | 4 | 5 | 6 | 7 | 8 | 9 | 10

On this scale

- a score of 10 represents a feeling of being 'absolutely full' of energy
- a score of 1, a feeling of being 'absolutely drained'
- scores of 2–9 represent the varying degrees of energy in between.

In the hope of getting a truer picture, we will ask our subjects to score their energy levels in this manner at six different time points throughout each day, and for seven consecutive days. At the end of the week we would collect all of the data and plot it on a graph. This is what we would find:

Graph 1. Energy levels of healthy people throughout a typical day

Absolutely full of energy	10
	9
Plenty of energy	8
	7
Good energy	6
	5
Poor energy	4
	3
	2
Absolutely drained of energy	1

8 a.m. 10 a.m. 12 a.m. 2 p.m. 4 p.m. 6 p.m. 10 p.m.

We can learn several things about the energy levels of our healthy friends from this graph:

1. Energy levels clearly fluctuate throughout the day.
2. They are relatively good in the late morning.
3. They peak at midday (or thereabouts).
4. They gradually decline as the afternoon progresses.

Twenty per cent of healthy people enjoy a second burst of energy between the hours of eight and ten in the evening. These are mostly students — they should enjoy it while they can! One observation not shown on the graph is that many healthy people experience a transient dip in energy in the early afternoon, which some of them have discovered they can fend off with a cup of coffee. But, as you will see in Chapter 16, they wouldn't have this slump if they avoided caffeine in the first place! Meanwhile, have you noticed that the highest average score is only 70 per cent, and that much of the day is spent below optimum levels of energy? Now that's interesting! These people have specifically informed us that they are not feeling tired, but neither are they on top of the world. In fact, it is very rare to meet someone who is always bursting with energy. It would seem, therefore, that healthy individuals are content so long as they have sufficient energy to carry out their basic tasks with relative ease; and that brings us to another concept, namely, the perception of effort.

The perception of effort

We have already established that the feeling of fatigue is a subjective experience. As we turn our attention now to the sense of energy — the antithesis of fatigue — the first thing we have to say is that it too is a subjective feeling. Of course, from a scientific point of view, we understand that energy is defined as the capacity for work, and it can be measured in joules. You will see in Chapter 13 that the energy content of various foods can also be accurately measured (in calories). But with reference to our sense of well-being and our sense of vigour, the concept of energy is more difficult to define. It is best understood as a *perception* of the ease with which we can accomplish our normal activities.

People who feel that they can carry on through life with ease, fulfilling their various responsibilities and enjoying their pastimes, do not complain of fatigue. Their perception of effort is low; they have plenty of energy. The fatigued, on the other hand, have a variable perception of effort. Some may be able to function fairly well in terms of their responsibilities, their 'obligatory activities', as it were. But there is always a cost. They have to speak to themselves, motivate themselves and even consciously force themselves to do what needs to be done. They no longer engage in what they now consider to be luxury activities, such as hobbies or a social life. Others, more severely affected, simply cannot muster the energy required for even the most basic daily tasks. Let me give you one simple example of this. When healthy people stand at the foot of the stairs, they look up, see a few steps and take them two by two; those with chronic debilitating fatigue look up, see Mount Everest, and sigh.

So where does our perception of effort come from? Where is our sense of energy? We have a respiratory centre in the brain, along with a speech centre, a motor cortex, a sensory cortex, and even a pleasure centre. So do we have an energy centre? No. There is no single energy centre in the brain. Rather, the perception of energy is the end product of several interacting factors, all equally important. These can be considered under two headings: physiological (body) and psychological (mind). Our bodies may be primarily healthy or diseased, fit or unfit, well nourished or malnourished etc. The sum total of these will make up our physiological status, and this in turn will determine the sort of messages that are sent to our conscious brain. We will feel well or unwell, or somewhere in between. However, these feelings of wellness are interpreted and influenced by other factors, namely, our psychological make-up and our social surroundings.

We have learned much about the psychological influences on our perception of effort/energy from the field of sports psychology. Think of it this way: an athlete completes a 1,500 metre race in a time of 3m. 48.58; he says he went flat out, gave it everything he had and couldn't have run any faster. But why not? What prevented him from completing the same distance one second faster, or even one-tenth of a second faster? This may seem like a banal question to the fatigued, but elite athletes would love to find the answer. They are well aware that medals can be decided on the basis of a split second. Obviously the answer to the question has a lot to do with physical ability and fitness, but there is much more to the story: there is a perception of effort involved. Even when he was still in the dressing room, our runner was anticipating the amount of effort that would be required of him to win, and he approached his race with some degree of confidence and/or trepidation. As he set off with the sound of the starter's gun, he knew he had to run a full 1,500 metre race. He had to pace himself, conserve energy and yet expend it. He also had tactical considerations. Was he up against a fast finisher? Should he set the pace or stay with the pack? He would have had a game plan to start with, but what would happen to his confidence if an opponent made an early break? What should he do, stay with him or hang back? Furthermore, perhaps our runner was aware that the national coach was watching his performance, with a view to a place on the team.

As you can see, many diverse influences are at play here, both internal and external. These are what psychologists call dispositional (personality) and situational factors respectively, and they assure us that our personalities account for up to 80 per cent of our perception of effort. Isn't that staggering? What they have found is that the extrovert, confident and hard driven, who feel in control of their circumstances and who tend to minimise their discomfort, are likely to report low perceptions of effort. These are the so called type A personalities. They suppress their feelings of fatigue, they are time conscious and they frequently need to be in charge of their surroundings.They cannot allow themselves to feel their fatigue, for to do so would interfere with their need for mastery. They pay a high price for this, however, because they can be difficult to get along with, and they are at increased risk of heart disease. Conversely, those who are introvert, passive and lacking in self-confidence, who feel they are controlled by their circumstances rather than being in control, and who tend to care about their discomfort, experience higher perceptions of effort. Remember we are talking here about the super fit, not just the fatigued.

Come back for a moment to our athlete. What would have been required of him to run one-tenth of a second faster? We can work this out mathematically: he would have to increase his effort by a factor of less than 0.05 per cent — not a lot, but a noticeable difference. What he will aim for now, in future training, is to achieve this increase.

The idea of a 'just noticeable difference' is interesting, and not just for athletes. Whenever we are engaged in an activity, such as walking on a treadmill, we are conscious, to some extent at least, of the effort required to keep pace. But a sports psychologist could increase the speed of the treadmill ever so slightly without telling us, and we would fail to notice the difference. In other words, we would not perceive the increase in effort required.The speed could be further increased by several minute increments before we would perceive the increased effort. This is what is meant by a just noticeable difference.

The implication for the profoundly fatigued is that they too can increase their output by tiny increments without doing themselves any harm, and these increments in activity can be further increased ever so slightly as time goes by.We will address this in some detail in Chapter 25.

Energy levels in fatigue

So what about the fatigued? What happens to their perception of effort? To find out, we could ask them to complete the same energy graph, using the same rating scale and time frame as before.This is what we would find:

Graph 2. Energy levels of fatigued patients throughout a typical day

Absolutely full of energy	10		
	9		
Plenty of energy	8		
	7		Healthy
Good energy	6		
	5		
Poor energy	4		
	3		
	2		Fatigued
Absolutely drained of energy	1		

8 a.m. 10 a.m. 12 a.m. 2 p.m. 4 p.m. 6 p.m. 10 p.m.

As expected, fatigue patients have lower energy levels than normal. Furthermore, 75 per cent of them experience a profound slump in energy as they progress through the afternoon. These are the ones who have to drag themselves through the day with ever dwindling supplies of energy. By evening time they are completely washed out and fit only for bed. There are several other insights to be gleaned from this graph:

1. Patients with chronic fatigue also experience fluctuating energy levels throughout the course of a day.
2. Their best hours are usually in the mid to late morning.
3. Their energy peaks a midday (or thereabouts).

These findings are important to fatigued individuals. In the first place, it is very rare to find a patient who is *totally* debilitated *all* the time. Even the very ill have a little respite at some point in the day. They may feel tired all day long, but there is a window of opportunity, so to speak, during which they can fulfil at least some of their responsibilities and other activities (more on this in Chapter 25).

While we are on the subject, I would like to say something else about the nature of fatigue. Fatigue is usually a 'central' symptom, not a 'peripheral' one. Let me explain. Central, in this context, refers to the central nervous system, and specifically to the brain. Peripheral refers to everything else, but specifically to the muscles in our limbs. After all, these are what we use to accomplish the functional activities of everyday life. Research into the muscular function of patients with chronic fatigue suggests that their muscles are basically healthy! They are, admittedly, out of condition, but formal assessments of muscle strength are often normal. Having said that, there is a suggestion that fatigued muscles fail to contract to their maximum, and that muscular activity leads to inappropriate biochemical and cardiac responses in the fatigued patient. This implies that there is central interference with muscular function.

We have paid homage to the importance of psychological influences on our perception of effort (and fatigue), and we will cover this extensively in the next section; but the central interference referred to here is much more than a question of psychology or motivation. Please understand this: there is a fundamental change in the day-to-day running of the fatigued brain. Simply put, the automatic functions we all take for granted (such as running up the stairs) are no longer performed automatically and with ease. These activities must now be performed by supervised effort. In other words, the fatigued patient becomes conscious of unconscious activity. This is the basis of the increased sense of effort experienced by the fatigued.

It is interesting to note that all people (healthy, tired and very tired) experience daily fluctuations in energy levels. It is equally interesting to observe the associations that exist between energy and mood. If we asked our healthy subjects to rate their mood as 'good', 'fair' or 'bad' along with their energy levels, we would discover that good mood coincides with higher energy levels. The fatigued patients would report a similar pattern. But we would find no association, in either group, between low mood and poor energy. I know this is a little complicated, but take my word for it, this provides evidence of the *physiological* (not psychological) basis of both of these distinct human experiences. It has to do with our 'internal body clock' — our circadian rhythm (page 77).

As a final thought, what happens to the perception of effort in those who feel they have completely or almost completely recovered from their fatigue? Well, as expected, they have higher energy levels than those who are still suffering. But, surprisingly and in spite of obvious satisfaction with their own progress, some of them may still score below normal. In other words, they still have a higher perception of effort. This is further evidence that chronic fatigue is primarily a disturbance of our perception of effort; and it suggests that the worst affected patients may find it hard to shake off the remnants of this perception, even when they are improving in every other respect. A solution to this dilemma is offered in Chapter 25.

Section 2

The Most Common Causes of Fatigue

(I) PSYCHOLOGICAL AND PSYCHIATRIC EXPLANATIONS OF FATIGUE

(II) PHYSICAL EXPLANATIONS OF FATIGUE

Social Attitudes to Psychological Distress

3

In Chapter 1 we followed 100 hypothetical patients whose chief complaint was one of chronic fatigue. We saw that 70 per cent of these would eventually and correctly be given a psychiatric diagnosis. In descending order of frequency, the main problems identified were depression, anxiety, panic, phobia and somatisation. Because they are so important in the evaluation of fatigue, each of these will be examined in this section. Stress, which is so frequently associated with depression, will also be covered. But before we get into the details, let us voice the question that we are all dying to ask. How can patients complaining of fatigue end up with a psychiatric diagnosis? We have clearly stated that they presented themselves as tired; they sought help for fatigue, not depression or anxiety. Neither did they complain of phobic fear. So, you may well ask, what's going on?

There are several possible explanations for this. In the first place, fatigue may be the covert forerunner of depression. In other words, it may be the only feeling that a patient is aware of at the onset of a depressive illness. These patients are not trying to hide their depressed mood. In fact, they will tell us that they are not feeling depressed — not yet. As time goes by, however, the mood will begin to fall. This is what happens. The chemicals (neurotransmitters) in the brain responsible for mood are also involved in our sense of 'energy'. If these chemicals are in short supply, the patient starts to feel tired, and may feel no other symptom. As levels fall further, the mood begins to droop, and eventually all the salient features of a depressive illness will become manifest.

Another reason for the masquerading of psychiatric illness as fatigue is that we as a society are still not comfortable with expressing our psychological distress. This is particularly true of us men. We are much happier discussing our physical ailments, and some of us even boast about these! We find it more comfortable to say, 'I feel tired' than to admit 'I feel sad and tearful.' We readily draw the doctor's attention to our physical ailments, but we skirt around the psychological issues. Ironically then, it is often our physical symptoms which prevent us from getting the psychological help we really need. We still think that psychiatric illness is a sign of weakness, some sort of failure on our part. It is not, and I hope this will become abundantly clear as you read through this chapter. This is important for all of us, because stress and depression — and how we cope with them — have far-reaching implications for health. Together they are the commonest causes of fatigue, and they give rise to a substantial number of other physical and mental symptoms.

Case history

Margaret is a 38-year-old housewife who asked me to visit her at home because she didn't have the energy to come to my office. She complained of extreme weakness and had been more or less bed-bound for the previous five weeks. She looked dishevelled, and the house was unkempt. 'I've no strength in my body at all', she said as she struggled down the hall towards her bedroom. She had been coping fairly well until a recent bout of flu. But by this she did not mean that she previously enjoyed full health. In fact, she hadn't really felt well for ages.

Her problems first started some twelve years ago, with the symptoms of an irritable bowel: bloating of the abdomen and colicky pains relieved by the passage of diarrhoeal stool. Shortly afterwards she had her first of many 'dizzy spells', and from this time on her energy levels were low. Over the next few years she suffered frequent bouts of sinusitis and urinary tract infections. These were treated with antibiotics. At one stage her doctor prescribed a tonic to try to impart some energy, but to no avail. She had to leave her job on account of the tiredness and the pains which had since started in her muscles. She reckons she would have been sacked anyway, as she was no longer able to cope with the workload. At this point her husband was unexpectedly made redundant, and she became very depressed. She found herself increasingly anxious and irritable, at times overwhelmed with a feeling of impending disaster. This feeling of dread regularly developed into full-blown panic attacks (see Chapter 6). Although she had considered herself as happily married, she and her husband had certain difficulties with their sexual relationship which had never been properly addressed.

This is clearly a very complicated picture. Irritable bowel has a food intolerance basis in at least 70 per cent of cases, but may also be aggravated by psychological influences. She has suffered recurrent infections over many years, and now has some features of postviral debility. The dizzy spells and panic attacks are hallmarks of anxiety, she has a sizeable psychosexual problem and she is undoubtedly depressed. Treatment must be directed at *all* these factors before we will see any improvement in her condition. It was some time before Margaret could admit that she needed psychological help. She was much more comfortable with the notion that she was 'only physically ill', and she could happily discuss her numerous physical symptoms in great detail and at some length. When she did eventually go for counselling, she made some real progress. She is now much better than when she was first seen, although she still has some way to go.

Margaret's attitude to the psychological aspects of illness is by no means unique. There is a great reluctance generally to accept any diagnosis which sounds remotely psychological or psychiatric in nature. I well remember the professor of psychiatry in my medical school lamenting this problem. He used to relate a story which epitomised his experience. He went out socially one evening with two of his colleagues, one a surgeon, the other a physician. He could see that their patients approached them quite happily: 'How nice to see you, Mrs Skilled Surgeon. I haven't even burped since you took out my gall bladder!' and 'How are you Dr Clever Fellow? My breathing has been perfect since you gave me that inhaler.' But the poor psychiatrist had no such joy. Although he recognised one or two of his patients in the crowd, they were invariably looking the other way. He was never acknowledged to be anybody's doctor. Not that they were ungrateful; on the contrary, they appreciated him very much, but they preferred to express their gratitude in the privacy of his consulting rooms where, as they hoped, nobody would see them come or go.

The stigma surrounding psychiatric illness and other psychological difficulties seems to emanate from a pernicious value judgment which goes something like this: you must be an altogether inferior person if you cannot cope on your own and have to call on a counsellor for help. We must completely reject and distance ourselves from such an attitude. The fact is that one out of seven people will seek the help of either a psychiatrist or psychologist at some stage in their lives. Many more will consult their family doctors with psychological troubles. That's a lot of people, and there are undoubtedly others who would benefit but never come forward. They are too afraid of what other people might think. Might not their friends think them weak, or look upon them as having some degree of impending madness? The fact is, people who need help for psychological problems are ordinary folk like you and me. They may have been pressed beyond measure into the doldrums of depression or some other psychological difficulty, but rather than sit back and suffer it, they want to do something about it. In seeking professional help, they are assuming full responsibility for themselves. They are exercising their freedom of choice to face up to the truth, resolve the relevant issues and grow into full-orbed human beings. Far from being in any way inferior, these are the brave ones who seek recovery and are willing to pay the price for it. The only attitude we can adopt in the face of such courage and determination is one of respect and admiration. A ready acceptance of our vulnerabilities as human beings will help us to acknowledge our stresses and admit to our feelings without the fear of judgment. It will also help us to empathise with those around us who are still suffering.

4 *Stress*

Stress, by definition, is our perception of and reaction to any life event that requires us to change. We are well aware of the difficulty of adverse life events, but stressful events are not necessarily unpleasant. In fact, any event that requires change can be perceived as stressful. A new job, a promotion at work, an inheritance, or even winning the national lottery may all be considered positive and pleasant experiences, but they all demand something of us. We have to cope with and adapt to our new circumstances. No two people are the same in this regard, so in order to understand the challenge that a given life event presents to a particular individual, we must first understand how they perceive and adapt to the event. It's how we think we can cope that's important, not whether we are right or wrong in our thinking. Our appraisal of the new challenge will determine our immediate reaction to it and our ability to adjust to it in the long term.

We are all, without exception, subject to stress. We are affected by the pressure of difficult life circumstances as and when they arise, and we carry within us the emotional pain of past events, together with the tension of the ongoing psychological problems which they have produced. Those who emerge battered and torn from childhood are left with a greater degree of emotional vulnerability than those more fortunate. They are more likely to be introspective and lacking in self-confidence (having a rather low opinion of themselves). Not surprisingly, they have no great hopes for their future. Those who escape from childhood without major trauma, and who are allowed to come into adult life from a stable and secure emotional background, enjoy a much healthier internal environment.

So, our ability to handle stress is determined, at least in part, by the inner strength of our psychological make-up. As we have seen, those who have been wounded may find it harder to cope. But whatever our background, we are still only human, and there is only so much that we can bear. The fact that we all have a breaking point has been clearly demonstrated by the experience of soldiers on the battle front. They are subject to great stress; they constantly face injury and death; they are weather beaten, sleep deprived and hungry. The sound of gunfire and the sight of falling comrades is a terrible agony. If not soon delivered from this awful predicament, even the bravest soldier will develop a crippling anxiety state called 'battle fatigue'. Almost all people, if exposed for long enough, will collapse in this way. Figures released by the US Army show that 75 per cent of soldiers can be expected to have broken down in this manner within 140 days of battle, and 90 per cent within 210 days. The British Army has had a similar experience in Northern Ireland, in that many of its soldiers have developed serious psychological problems whilst serving there. As you can see, there are not many who are invincible; nor are there many heroes.

It is clear, then, that the duration of a stressful event (e.g. the number of days in battle) has a bearing on our ability to cope. We are better able to handle stressful events of short duration. Take natural disasters, for instance. Twenty-five per cent of victims are able to keep going and to function well in the immediate aftermath of a major disaster. They are able to help other victims who may be in the throes of an acute stress reaction (shocked). Furthermore, once the immediate threat has passed, fewer than 25 per cent of all victims will suffer from post-traumatic stress.

These are, of course, extreme models of stress, but they do demonstrate some interesting principles which are relevant to our everyday lives, albeit on a smaller scale. Sometimes life is like a battlefield, a fight for survival, and it should come as no surprise that some of us become battle fatigued under its stresses. The strong may outlast the weak for a while, but they too are vulnerable, and they too can fall. Human nature is basically frail.

Case history

Michael was a successful man in his late forties. He was happily married with three lovely children, and very well off financially, with established business interests in a number of European countries. He enjoyed a wholesome childhood, coming from a farming background in which the family worked hard and learned to pull together. In the last few years, Michael ran into some difficult circumstances. His wife became ill with a nasty bowel disease which left her in a lot of pain. Michael, who obviously cared for her, could not bear to watch her suffering. After some time, he himself started to feel sick. He felt as if he wanted to vomit, although he never could. The persisting nausea was eventually overtaken by a low mood: he felt down in the dumps and his energy reserves fell to an all-time low. It was most unusual for him to feel sad — he had always been so capable and strong. But he now found himself increasingly depressed and worried. The stress had taken its toll.

We should not forget the enormous stress that falls on people like Michael, who care for their loved ones in times of long-term illness. A survey in the UK has revealed that two-thirds of those who care for sick family members at home will themselves become ill.

LEAGUE TABLE OF STRESSFUL EVENTS

We used to think of stressful events in terms of a 'league table', and we classified them according to our general perception of the difficulties they would present. Thus, we had categories ranging from catastrophic stress (e.g. the death of a child or the suicide of a spouse), through severe stress (e.g. getting divorced) and down to mild stress (e.g. a child leaving home). However, each individual will perceive stress differently. For example, a child leaving home may be a relief for some parents, but the end of the world for others. Having said that, most of us would agree on the following list of stresses:

- Bereavement
- Serious physical illness, major disasters, persecution
- Violent, physical or sexual assault, serious accident

- Divorce
- Separation
- Birth of a child (especially the first)
- Getting married
- Marital disharmony
- Moving (or building) house
- Problems with friends, neighbours or associates
- Parenting
- Financial pressures
- Legal problems
- Work-related stress: restructuring, evaluations, mergers, promotion, redundancy, role ambiguity, workload etc.
- Life-cycle transitions, ageing and imminent retirement
- Rapid social change
- Non-events may also be stressful (e.g. not receiving affection).

It stands to reason that a run of bad luck, in which several stressful events occur in rapid succession, would be more difficult to cope with than any single event (unless that event is life threatening, see below). In this sense, stress is cumulative. Medical studies confirm the greater incidence of illness among those who have been through several stresses, and we can now say with some degree of confidence that more stress leads to more illness. Another feature of stress is that we can become sensitised by it. Perhaps the clearest example of this is found in the experience of people who suffer from post-traumatic stress disorder (PTSD).

Case history

Peter, for instance, was a 52-year-old farmer who presented with complaints of chronic tiredness and generalised pains. His problem started some four years previously after he 'broke a few bones', he said. At first he only had pain at the site of his fractures, but then he developed widespread pain which persisted in spite of pain-killers. He also volunteered that his sleep pattern was disturbed. When I asked Peter about the accident that led to his injuries, he started shifting uncomfortably on his chair, a slight tremor appeared in his hands, he became short of breath and his forehead produced small beads of sweat. He was terrified. He was clearly reluctant to talk about his experience, but he eventually told me some of the details. One day during harvest his machinery broke down. He was leaning into the harvester, trying to find the problem, when the motor suddenly started up again. He was caught in the machine and severely injured as a result. He was stuck there, unable to move or to do anything to help himself, other than wait for someone to find and rescue him. He was lucky to get out alive, let alone with all his limbs. Having heard this story, I asked a few more pertinent questions. Following the incident, Peter admitted he had lost all interest in his farm, his life's work. He also had troublesome nightmares in which he relived the accident again and again. Not only that, but he had vivid pictures and thoughts of the accident flashing intrusively across his mind even during his waking hours. He was also cranky and very jumpy. He would startle at the slightest noise, often bolting upright from his armchair when the doorbell rang. We call this state hypervigilance. Peter is suffering from a post-traumatic stress disorder, in which he has become sensitised (hypervigilant) by his experience.

Once again this is an extreme model of stress. But people who go through difficult times, particularly if these are drawn out over prolonged periods of time, may also become sensitised in like manner.

Case history

Take Marilyn, for example. A few years ago she had one of those runs of bad luck that I mentioned above. One thing after another went wrong in her life. It got to the stage where she was just waiting for the next calamity. Towards the end of this period she developed a widespread itchy rash of hives. This eventually settled with treatment, but she has been prone to recurrent attacks on and off since then. She noticed that her rash was stress sensitive, i.e. it would likely come back when she was under pressure. What she couldn't figure out was why it would recur when the stress was minor, or even insignificant. The reason is that she has become sensitised. To put it simply, her skin is hypervigilant and over-reacts to mild stresses as if they were catastrophic.

THE PHYSICAL EFFECTS OF STRESS AND DEPRESSION

The relationship between stress and illness is undisputed. Stress increases the activity of our sympathetic nervous system — the nerves that automatically control our major bodily functions such as heart rate, blood pressure, breathing, intestinal motility etc. The adrenaline surge we experience when we get a fright, or when we are called upon to perform some unaccustomed task, leads to the well-known 'fight or flight' response. Stress also increases the activity of other hormones, and especially those that play a central role in our brain. Specifically, the hormones of the hypothalmic-pituitary-adrenal axis are activated, resulting in an increase in cortisol (steroid) levels. In due course and particularly if the stress is prolonged, alterations in neurotransmitters occur. Now our mood is at risk, our energy levels fall, our sleep quality suffers and we lose our appetite etc. This is the mechanism by which stress leads to depression. Notice that even though the stress may be a psychosocial one, the changes that occur in the body are physical (and they are amenable to physical treatment). In other words, depression is not just 'all in the mind'. It has a physical substrate, a biological vehicle of expression.

Sometimes the stress itself is a physical one. Viral infections, a major operation, an underactive thyroid gland or any other physical illness can all result in disturbed brain biochemistry. But whatever their origin, stress and depression have the power to wreak havoc. For instance, it has been known since antiquity that depressed women are more likely to develop cancer than their non-depressed friends. This disturbing observation was first made by Galen (A.D. 129–199), one of the great fathers of medicine, and his finding has been upheld by present-day researchers. These have not only confirmed the greater incidence of cancer in depressed patients of both sexes, but have further identified them as suffering from more allergies, more frequent infections and more auto-immune diseases than their happier counterparts. Needless to say, stress can also aggravate any pre-existing physical illness.

COPING WITH STRESS

Why is it then that two-thirds of carers (like Michael) become ill, and the other third do not? Why are 25 per cent of disaster victims able to cope better than their fellows? And why do 75 per cent of disaster victims escape the misery of PTSD, whilst the others do not? What protects these people from stress-related illness when they are under duress?

We have already seen that stress, and how we cope with it, affects our immune system; and that psychological make-up determines, at least in part, our susceptibility to infection, the duration of our illnesses and the severity of our allergies. It stands to reason that a robust mental health and an optimistic outlook on life confer some degree of protection against illness. We can take a closer look at this question of coping and, specifically, the coping strategies that seem to help. The hardy among us employ four main coping skills when faced with stress, and that's why they suffer less physical illness, less anxiety, less depression, and why they enjoy a longer life. These skills can be summarised as follows:

1. They gain as much control as they can over the stressful situation.
2. They are prepared to take the bull by the horns and get into the mode of problem-solving. They don't stick their head in the sand and hope it will go away. If necessary, they are prepared to forgo short-term pleasure for long-term gain.
3. They make healthy choices in relation to diet, exercise and relaxation.
4. They have developed and make use of social supports. They discuss their problems with family and friends.

5   *Depression*

Practically speaking, depression is almost always the result of stress. Even the diagnosis of so called 'endogenous depression' has fallen out of favour now; it was applied to those severe depressions which were thought to arise from a disturbance of brain function, regardless of any past or present life events. This was in contrast to 'reactive depression', which was seen to arise directly from difficult life circumstances. It is now widely held that all depression is a reaction to some underlying physical or psychological stress.

It may not be easy to identify the psychological contribution to a depressed state when it is hidden among unpleasant and painful childhood experiences, but in the majority of cases, gentle and careful questioning by a skilled counsellor will eventually uncover the root. This holds true, not just for the so called 'neurotic' depressions, but for the severely psychotic types as well, in which the patient's mind is filled with paranoia or other such delusions. This explains why psychotherapy is often an effective therapy in the management of depression.

Physical factors also predispose an individual to depression. Genetic inheritance (family history) and biochemical (mood neurotransmitter) abnormalities in the brain leave some individuals even more susceptible to the depressive effects of their stresses. Furthermore, depression often occurs in the absence of any psychological trigger. It's been said before but it's worth repeating: depression is not all in the mind. For example, the patient who develops an underactive thyroid gland may present to the doctor with a depressed mood, and little else. This depression will respond fully and dramatically to thyroid hormone replacement. So, was that depression psychological or physical? Physical, of course! And there are many other examples of this sort in medical practice — so much so that a doctor will not accept a diagnosis of depression without first checking for a physical root. Why then are we still so reluctant as a society to face up to this?

Case history

One example of physical depression that clearly sticks out in my mind is that of a successful bank manager who was admitted to a psychiatric ward during my training days. He had no reason to be depressed: he was happily married with healthy kids, sufficient money, and was doing well at work etc. Then one day he saw little ghouls messing about in his back garden! Having observed them for several nights, he became convinced they were plotting to destroy him, so he stayed up all night to make sure they would not succeed. By the time he was admitted to hospital he could hardly talk. Every word was painfully laboured and took an age to articulate, and his physical movement was extremely sluggish. He had a severe depressive illness with psychotic features. Then I met his wife. The contrast was staggering. She was bright and cheerful, and not at all worried. I was puzzled by this. Did she not understand how ill her husband was? 'Oh I do, doctor, but sure he's been here before! And I'm sure he'll get better again.' She was referring to a previous bout of depression which was almost identical to this one, *some ten years earlier.* At that time he was admitted in much the same state as he was now and responded dramatically to treatment. He went back to his family and to his job, and had led a normal and fulfilling life in the interim. I could hardly believe it, but sure enough, he responded to treatment within a matter of weeks and was discharged home in his right mind, hopefully to enjoy (at least) another ten years of good mental health.

Needless to say, this patient had a very severe illness (the vast majority of depressed patients are not nearly as bad as this). Psychotic features are fortunately rare in depression. But the point is that severe as well as mild depressions may have a physical base.

The many faces of depression

Depression, when it is severe enough to cause unremitting fatigue, refers not merely to the periods of sadness which we all experience from time to time, but to a clinical syndrome characterised by a serious and sustained collapse of mood which doctors call a 'depressive illness'. When they present openly, depressed patients are easily recognised: they weep and look dejected; they lose interest in their appearance and food; they complain of poor concentration and forgetfullness, of anxiety and irritability, of weakness and fatigue. They report sleepless nights and troubled minds. They cannot find pleasure in any pursuit. Feelings of guilt and despair are often expressed and, as life loses its appeal, these may develop into suicidal proportions. Various physical symptoms accompany the mental ones, but the patient, relatives and doctor all agree upon the diagnosis of depression and upon the need for treatment.

However, depression does not always declare itself so plainly. We have already seen how some of us focus more on our bodily symptoms than on our minds and hearts. These patients will attend the doctor complaining of headache on one day and constipation the next; of 'queer feelings all over' one week and painful limbs the next; of double vision one month and fatigue the next. They are often extensively investigated by one medical specialist after another. All the tests are normal, of course, but instead of bringing comfort, this paradoxically only serves to heighten anxiety: the patient may continue to believe that he has cancer or some other serious malady which the physician has not yet discovered. A patient in this condition may become completely preoccupied with himself, and every minor, mysterious symptom assumes enormous importance (another kind of hypervigilance). Brave counsellors will now try to divert attention away from the loud physical complaints and seek to identify the real psychological state which underlies them. Are there problems at home, with the kids, or in the marriage? What about the situation at work? Are you under financial pressure? Is there a sexual difficulty of some sort? What was your childhood like anyway? But the hypochondriac (for that's what he is called) adamantly denies that stress or depression has anything to do with his complaint, and any suggestion to the contrary is met with an angry, hostile reaction. We do not accuse him of lies or of hysteria. We acknowledge that he has very real symptoms, but we contend that there is nothing wrong with him physically. If at last he can be persuaded to accept this and adopt the psychological approach, he will receive appropriate counselling and hopefully find lasting relief.

Further confusion may arise when depression takes on the very clever disguise of a smile. The 'smiling depressive', as he is known in the trade, is perhaps the most difficult to identify. In spite of having many of the symptoms listed above, he maintains a pleasant and jolly appearance. He does not come across as being particularly worried about his symptoms; nor is he angry with his doctor when no explanation is forthcoming. He too will flatly deny a low mood, and unless an astute doctor can pick him out, he will be subjected to the same merry-go-round of endless, unnecessary investigations. It may seem unbelievable that such a contradiction as smiling depression exists, but the proof that it does is in the successful restoration of such patients to full health when appropriate counselling and/or antidepressant treatment is given.

When is sadness depression?

Admittedly, it can be difficult to draw the line between what should be allowed as 'normal' sadness and when it becomes 'abnormal'. For example, who would deny the right of the bereaved to weep, or to express feelings of loss and despair? We almost expect them to withdraw from society somewhat, and to want to be alone for a while. We understand why they go off their food and lose weight, and why they cannot sleep. They are grieving. But if they are still withdrawn five years later, or if they feel so depressed as to contemplate suicide, then we would have to draw the line and offer some sort of intervention. The diagnosis of a depressive illness that needs treatment is therefore based on an assessment of the severity and duration of symptoms.

Fatigued or depressed?

The question of whether stress and depression are the cause of a patient's symptoms, or the result of them, is not always easy to answer. This applies to fatigue as well as to any other symptom.

Depressed patients will invariably complain of feeling tired. It is part and parcel of their overall lethargic condition. Fatigued patients, on the other hand, may or may not be depressed. Those who are not are able to enjoy themselves as much as their energy levels allow. Their interest in life is maintained and they get on with it as best they can. It is a source of great frustration to these patients when neither their doctors nor their families believe them to be anything other than depressed. Those who do become depressed do so because of the frustrating limitations imposed on them by their fatigue. This should be a perfectly understandable reaction to what is, after all, a debilitating symptom, but it continues to be the focal point of contention: are you depressed because you are fatigued, or are you fatigued because, underneath it all, you are really depressed? Patients frequently find themselves arguing over this point with their doctors, and the doctor-patient relationship will become increasingly strained if no agreement is reached. Indeed, some previously good relationships have come to total ruin in these controversial waters.

In practice, it does not matter whether the depression (if it is there) came first or second. The point is, if it is present at all, it needs to be acknowledged as such and explored. It may be difficult to distinguish between physical and psychosomatic symptoms initially, but the true origins of each should become apparent as time goes by. With this in mind, it may be wise to withhold judgment at the start of treatment until the truth becomes clear.

Case history

Caroline first came to see me at the age of 23. She complained mostly of fatigue, but she had a host of other symptoms as well: poor concentration, dizziness, bloating of the abdomen, headache, joint pains and mood swings. These symptoms began five years ago, shortly after she had started a new job, and they were getting progressively worse. We embarked on a course of treatment which was aimed primarily at the troublesome physical complaints, believing the mood swings to be a reaction to these. At each visit we got to know each other a little better.

She had been fairly happy as a child, doted upon by devoted

parents who were exceedingly proud of their little girl. Having had no other children, they took a special interest in every detail of Caroline's life. Unfortunately, they went overboard and made meddlesome decisions on her behalf; they even chose her (I-know-what's-best-for-you) career. It's not as if she was stupid or anything. She had been successful at school and would have been quite capable of making that decision, but they did not allow her time to explore her own feelings or make her own decisions. She was not particularly ambitious for herself in the new job, but she felt under pressure from her parents to do well and to get places.

Her parents were concerned at the growing number of symptoms which she developed after she left home, but she never felt free to discuss what was really bothering her, namely, the growing feelings of anger and despair which were eating away at her on the inside. They would not listen; she knew this from bitter experience.

She married a very confident and successful businessman, and she was happy enough for a while. She then became unwell with abdominal symptoms, and the depression followed shortly afterwards. At one stage she held a bottle of pills in her hand and thought long and hard about an overdose. It would have ended all her problems; but she didn't really want to die, she just wanted to live differently! She felt as if she was of no use to anybody: 'I feel utterly inadequate', she said, after one year of regular visits to my office. That's how long it took. But even as the words were coming out of her mouth, she realised that she had hit the nail on the head: she felt *utterly inadequate*. She could then relate most of her present physical symptoms to that awful feeling, and she began to understand where it had come from.

Am I depressed?

Those who are suffering from fatigue need to ask themselves this question, and not least because depression is a treatable disorder. The following table contains a list of the principal symptoms of major depression. Ask yourself, over the last two weeks (or longer) have you had

Yes = 1
No = 0

1. Pervasive feelings of low mood.	
2. Loss of interest and/or pleasure in most activities.	

3. Loss of appetite (and weight) or over-eating (and weight gain).	
4. Insomnia or hypersomnia.	
5. Psychomotor retardation: movement and speech are very slow, or psychomotor agitation: constantly restless and agitated, pacing, unable to sit.	
6. Fatigue: this may be profound and debilitating. Simple activities may be very difficult to perform.	
7. Feelings of worthlessness and guilt.	
8. Difficulty concentrating and making decisions.	
9. Recurrent thoughts of death, with or without a plan for suicide.	
Score	/9

If you have ticked either 1 or 2 (or both), and have a total score of five (or more), you are suffering from major depression. Clearly, if you are feeling depressed but haven't scored five points, you would still be well advised to consult your doctor for a chat. You may well have a less severe form of the illness. There are other mood disorders, of course, and these may present differently. For example, atypical (unusual) depression is characterised by depressed mood together with increased appetite and weight gain, hypersomnolence, a feeling of leaden paralysis, and hypersensitivity to rejection.

Beware the diagnostic dump

Doctors are familiar with the various disguises of depression mentioned above — they deal with them regularly. They are also well aware of how easily psychological problems can cause physical complaints. It is for this reason that they so readily think along psychological lines when faced with symptoms which defy objective clinical or laboratory confirmation, particularly when these are accompanied by some alteration in mood. We must agree that they are often justified in doing so. Notwithstanding this, and in spite of what we have just discussed about the difficulty surrounding the diagnosis of depression, it is imperative that physical symptoms should not be attributed to stress or depression unless and until these can be positively identified as relevant to the case. Otherwise there is a danger that they will become some sort of 'dumping ground diagnosis' into which patients with baffling symptoms are cast by their frustrated doctors. Some patients feel that this has already happened, and the view that they now have of the medical profession, from the vantage point of this diagnostic dump, is not a pretty one. They are quite fed up of being dismissed as depressed or stressed when they know well they are not. They have fallen foul of the most common mistake in medicine — the assumption of psychological illness in the absence of physical signs of disease.

Case history

Mrs Campbell presented with a four year history of debilitating fatigue. She had been a keen gardener all her life, but was no longer able to follow her much-loved hobby on account of the tiredness. Her house, which she had always kept so proudly, was proving too hard to manage. She was 83 years old, but she was adamant that her symptoms had nothing to do with her great age. Her mind was in perfect working order, she was still driving her car, and she wanted to get back to her regular game of golf! She had been told that her fatigue was due to depression, but the fact that she had always been a happy-go-lucky person made her reject this diagnosis out of hand. Besides, she didn't even know what it was like to feel depressed. Nevertheless, she tried the antidepressants which her doctor prescribed — she would have tried anything — but the side effects were awful, so she abandoned this course of action. When a detailed enquiry was made into the precise circumstances surrounding the onset of her symptoms, something very interesting came to light. It turns out that she had been perfectly well up until she contracted a severe viral infection which required a hospital admission. Although the acute symptoms subsided within a few weeks, she never really recovered full strength afterwards. With this in mind, she was tentatively diagnosed as suffering from a postviral fatigue syndrome and treated appropriately. Within two short months of treatment she felt a vast improvement (see Chapter 22).

Anxiety, Panic and Phobia

6

Once again we must start by stating the obvious. Firstly, we all know what it's like to feel anxious and, secondly, anxiety is a very useful emotion. It is designed to protect us, or rather to ensure that we protect ourselves from harm. When faced with a threat we either stand our ground (and fight), or we turn and run (flight). Anxiety also helps us to prepare for important events, such as an interview or an exam. If we are not sufficiently anxious in our preparation and performance, we will not perform well. Similarly, we will also perform poorly if we are over-anxious. The secret of anxiety, then, is to have just the right amount of it, not too little and not too much. This section is for those among us who have too much. If you are one of these, the first thing to realise is that you are not alone: 5 per cent of the population suffers from a severe form of anxiety that substantially interferes with their quality of life. Women are affected more often than men, but this difference is not all that great.

Case history

Martin was in his early fifties when I first met him. He was well acquainted with the medical profession because he had consulted one doctor after another over many years. He was concerned about a number of symptoms, and he was hoping that I would be able to help where others had failed. I couldn't. In the first place he was worried. He also felt tired all the time. And then he complained of a host of other symptoms, including a racing heart, tightness in his chest, weakness in his legs, tingling in his hands and feet, and a gagging sensation in his mouth. He also volunteered that he was prone to panic attacks in certain stressful situations. It was clear that Martin was suffering from what doctors call a generalised anxiety disorder, in his case with panic attacks. The reason I couldn't help him was that he had trouble accepting this diagnosis — as much trouble taking it from me as from every other doctor he had consulted previously. He acknowledged that he was worried, of course, but he could not accept the fact that his tiredness and his other symptoms were related to his anxiety. But they were.

The classical feature of generalised anxiety disorder is worry, or anxiety. These are not the ordinary worries of everyday life which we all have from time to time. In health, we are able to control our worries, put them into perspective and take steps to deal with them. In generalised anxiety disorder (GAD) the worries are much more difficult to control. The focus of anxiety may be such common things as family safety, children's health, finances, performance at work, and the jobs that need doing etc. but the burden of worry in GAD is distressing and incapacitating. Life becomes laden with apprehension, a fear of imminent bad news. In addition to worry/anxiety, there are a number of other symptoms present, notably fatigue. For this reason, those who suffer from debilitating fatigue need to consider the possibility of GAD.

Am I anxious?

To help you answer this question, why not score yourself on the anxiety scale below. Over the past six months (or longer) have you experienced any of the symptoms shown there?

If you have answered yes to 1 and 2 on the anxiety sclae and if you have a total score of five (or more), then you are suffering from GAD. If you are feeling anxious but have not reached a total score of five, it could still be worth your while discussing this with your doctor or with a psychologist. You will have noticed that some of the symptoms of GAD overlap with those of depression. This is because depression is usually accompanied by some degree of anxiety. GAD, on the other hand, does not have a substantial depressive element. However, anxiety may occur in conjunction with panic attacks and/or phobias. Let's take a look at panic first. The short story opposite illustrates the process.

1. Pervasive feelings of worry or anxiety.	
2. Difficulty controlling your worries.	

3. Feelings of being on edge, restless.	
4. Fatigue.	
5. Difficulty with concentration, losing the thread of thought, mind going blank.	
6. Irritable cranky mood.	
7. Muscular tension and pain.	
8. Disturbed sleeping pattern: either insomnia or fitful non-refreshing sleep.	
Score	/8

Panic

She had always been a bit of a worrier, and she had never wanted to fly in the first place. She didn't like the thought of being up there in the sky, strapped to a seat in a cramped cabin, surrounded by people she didn't know. She had tried to calm her nerves with a drink before leaving home, but she was too nauseated and she felt quite bloated in the stomach. As she hoisted her suitcase on to the weighing scales at the check-in desk, an unusual heaviness came over her chest. She sighed deeply, trying to lift the sensation, but she obtained no relief. It made her feel a little caught for breath, so she sighed again, and then again. Her discomfort and apprehension grew as she sat waiting stiffly on the edge of her chair in the busy departure lounge. There were people everywhere, smiling and chatting confidently among themselves. She didn't feel a part of this strange scene; in fact, everything seemed distant to her, and so unreal. It was as if she was dreaming, as if she wasn't there at all. The other passengers seemed oblivious to her anxiety, and they were certainly unaware of the gathering storm within her. Her uneasy thoughts were interrupted by the sound of her flight number echoing across the hall. She jumped nervously to her feet, but as soon as she did, her head reeled in a dizzy swirl. She thought she might faint, so she sat down again for a moment to regain some composure. After a while she cautiously rose to her feet again and slowly made her way to the waiting aircraft, the inside of which was even smaller than she had expected. Her trembling and sweaty hands could not cope with the seat belt, so a stewardess with a reassuring but ineffective smile helped her. The aeroplane taxied out to the runway, paused for a few seconds, and then hurtled along at speed to become airborne. She felt cold and clammy all over, her heart was beating feverishly, and her head was splitting with pain. She looked out of the window at the shrinking landscape, but could focus on nothing. Her vision was blurred — she couldn't even read the emergency leaflet. She became increasingly agitated by her symptoms and suspected that they were serious, perhaps even terribly serious. The very thought further tightened her chest, and this made her breathing even more laboured than before. She was panting rapidly now, her lips and tongue were numb, her fingers tingled furiously, and she felt a threatening constriction in her throat. Finally, when she could no longer contain the unspeakable fear that gripped her, she cried out in agony for help and struggled desperately to release the confining seat belt. Startled faces turned curiously to see what all the commotion was about. She fell to the floor in great distress, totally out of control, screaming and shouting something about not being able to breathe. She was absolutely petrified. She thought she was going to die. The stewardess quickly placed a paper bag over the woman's mouth and nose, and asked her to blow into it. 'That's it. Nice and slowly now, breathe in — and out — breathe in — and out. That's good. You're doing fine.' At first the gasping passenger fought against the makeshift mask, but within a few minutes she felt the better for it. She was quickly relieved of her worst symptoms, and she managed to endure the rest of her flight, albeit with a thumping headache, by using the paper bag whenever she felt the need. This had been her first panic attack; she hoped it would be her last.

Panic and breathing

To understand what happens during a panic attack, we must first understand a little about breathing. Breathing is simply the mechanism whereby life-giving oxygen is delivered to cells, and the waste product, carbon dioxide, is taken from them. Firstly, air is drawn into the lungs. Oxygen then passes from the air into the blood and is transported in the red blood cells to every other cell in the body. Each cell then uses the oxygen to carry out its vital functions. Carbon dioxide is produced in the process as a waste product. The red cells, which have given the cell its oxygen, now gather up all the carbon dioxide and transport it back to the lungs. Here it is literally 'blown out' of the body. But carbon dioxide is far more than just a waste product. It plays a very important role in maintaining the chemical (acid-base) balance of the blood. The acid-base balance is of fundamental importance to the proper functioning of every cell in the body, and it is kept at a remarkably constant level by a symphony of 'buffer systems'. If the blood becomes too acidic, carbon dioxide mops up the excess acid; if it becomes too alkaline, carbon dioxide helps to make it more acidic. In this 'safety valve' manner, the acidity of blood is maintained at an optimum level for health.

Apart from buffer systems in the blood, there are two other major controls over blood chemistry: the kidneys, which are able to excrete acidic or alkaline urine; and the lungs, which exert their influence over blood chemistry by blowing off greater or lesser amounts of carbon dioxide. The more you breathe, the more carbon dioxide you get rid of. This will lower the blood level of carbon dioxide and render it more alkaline. The less you breathe, the more carbon dioxide you retain. This will elevate the blood level of carbon dioxide and render it more acidic.

In health, the breathing pattern is determined by a group of specialised cells in the brain, known as the respiratory centre. They are responsible for regulating the speed and depth of breathing. At rest, breathing is slow and shallow; during exercise it increases in speed and depth, always keeping pace with demand. The respiratory centre knows when to breathe fast and when to slow down, by measuring the level of carbon dioxide and the amount of acid in the blood. During exercise, carbon dioxide production increases dramatically and the respiratory centre responds by increasing the speed and depth of breathing. This allows all the excess carbon dioxide to be 'blown out' of the body, thus restoring chemical balance to the blood. As the level of carbon dioxide returns to the normal range, the respiratory centre correspondingly reduces the speed and depth of breathing. Thus, blood chemistry is stabilised by an appropriate breathing pattern.

Abnormal breathing

The increased speed and depth of breathing which occurs in response to high levels of carbon dioxide are entirely justified. But major problems arise from a breathing pattern which is inappropriately fast or deep, such as occurs in hyperventilation.

Imagine for a moment what would happen if the respiratory centre failed to slow the breathing rate after exercise. The carbon dioxide level would return to normal within a relatively short time, but continued fast breathing would make the lungs blow out more and more carbon dioxide from the body. This would result in an excessive loss of carbon dioxide, and the blood level of carbon dioxide would be abnormally low. This is called hypocapnia. The blood vessels which supply the brain are sensitive to hypocapnia, and they react to it by 'vasoconstriction', that is, they shut themselves down and deprive the brain of its full quota of blood in the process. The paradox of this situation then is that the brain is underoxygenated during episodes of over-breathing. An oxygen-starved brain is manifestly unhappy and makes its protest known through feelings of breathlessness, light-headedness, dizziness, blurring of vision and the occasional faint. In hypocapnia other chemical changes occur in the blood as a sort of knock-on effect: firstly, it becomes more alkaline (alkalosis); and secondly, the level of inorganic phosphorus falls (hypophosphataemia). Between them, these chemical changes give rise to a host of other symptoms including fatigue, malaise, pins and needles, numbness, headache, palpitations, chest pains, painful muscular spasms and bloating of the abdomen; and mental symptoms such as disorientation, feelings of unreality, anxiety and depression.

Acute hyperventilation — the panic attack

Panic attacks are usually an emotional response to stress. Sometimes the perceived threat (the trigger) is immediately obvious, but it may have its roots in life events long since forgotten. In these cases, patients may not be aware of why it is they feel panic.

Sometimes the trigger is a very specific phobia. These are pathological fears which lead the sufferer to avoidant behaviour, i.e. they avoid contact with the feared object or situation at all costs. The most common phobia is agoraphobia, a fear of being out alone in public places (such as walking, travelling, or in situations where one is likely to meet crowds). Agoraphobic individuals are sometimes able to manage an outing, but it will be with great discomfort, and they could start to panic if they feel they cannot escape. When agoraphobia is so severe as to limit all social contact, it is called a social phobia. This is another diagnosis for you to consider if you complain of debilitating fatigue. Does your fatigue prevent you from social contact? Strive at all times to maintain your social relationships, no matter how severe the fatigue. Refusal to do so raises the possibility of social phobia masquerading as fatigue.

Another well-known phobia is claustrophobia, a fear of enclosed spaces. For example, the claustrophobic will always use the stairs and avoid the elevator for fear of being trapped therein. Phobias may also be specifically confined to certain objects, such as a fear of spiders (arachnophobia) or needles (trephinophobia) or such like. Some phobias may develop from traumatic experiences. If you were bitten by a dog, for instance, you would naturally be wary of dogs for a while thereafter — that's normal enough. But if you developed a dog phobia, you would go to great lengths to avoid contact with dogs, or even the possibility of seeing a dog. It's the avoidant behaviour that characterises the phobia, together with the extreme anxiety generated by contact when it does occur, often to the point of a panic attack.

In any case, the panic subject responds to the trigger (whatever it may be) by breathing faster. They have a feeling of intense discomfort and uneasy anticipation. This may increase, crescendo fashion, to a feeling of impending doom or sheer terror. The increased breathing rate that follows this build-up of anxiety is inappropriate, and all the chemical changes of hyperventilation (outlined above) will ensue. The physical symptoms which follow are bizarre and frightening, and may themselves generate further anxiety — and hyperventilation. Patients in the throes of a panic attack often fear they are at death's door. In this sense, panic attacks are self-perpetuating. The attacks are also accompanied by the physical manifestations of anxiety, including rapid pulse, palpitations (abnormal heartbeat), dry mouth, nausea, sweating and headache etc. The patient is unaware of it, but the blood pressure goes up and the pupils dilate (causing blurred vision).

Have I ever had a panic attack?

Perhaps you have had one or more frightening experiences yourself and you wonder whether these represent episodes of panic. Compare your experience(s) with the following 'official criteria' for the diagnosis of panic attacks:

Yes = 1 No = 0

1. A sudden experience of intense fear or discomfort, followed within minutes by any four (or more) of the following symptoms:	
2. Palpitations	
3. Sweating	
4. Tremor	
5. Difficulty breathing	
6. Choking sensation	
7. Chest pain or tightness	
8. Nausea or other abdominal symptoms	
9. Dizziness or faint	
10. Feelings of unreality or detachment	
11. Fear of losing your mind or control	
12. Feeling you might die	
13. Pins and needles	
14. Going hot or cold	
Score	/14

If you have answered yes to 1 above, and if you have a total score of five or more, then you probably did have a panic attack.

Anxiety and chronic hyperventilation

Chronic anxiety may lead to chronic hyperventilation, an abnormal breathing pattern characterised by inappropriately fast and/or deep respirations over time. This over-breathing is not as dramatic as the acute hyperventilation of a panic attack, but it too may cause a number of chemical changes in the blood, and these in turn may give rise to symptoms, including fatigue. This is how it works. The abnormal breathing pattern of chronic anxiety leads to a permanently low level of carbon dioxide in the blood. After a while the respiratory centre begins to think of this low level as normal, and then strives to maintain it at all times. It has now learned a bad habit. The suffering patient is usually unaware of over-breathing because it is directed from the subconscious plane of the respiratory centre. Besides, when the blood is permanently hypocapnic, it only takes an occasional deep breath, or even a sigh, to keep it there. Thus, it is a state which is easy to maintain without any obvious outward sign of over-breathing. For this reason, this aspect of anxiety is often missed.

Case history

Steven is a 35-five-year-old computer engineer. He told me about his debilitating fatigue, which had started nine years previously and which was getting progressively worse as the years went by. He now felt completely drained of energy and was close to resigning from his job. In addition, he complained of weight loss, twitching muscles, abdominal discomfort, dull headaches, pins and needles in the hands and numbness in the legs. He thought his symptoms were made worse by certain foods, so he wondered if all his problems were food allergic in origin. As it turned out, they were not. The pins and needles, together with the other symptoms which he complained of, pointed to the possibility that he was anxious and hyperventilating. Steven was taught a simple, corrective breathing exercise. He performed this on a daily basis at home, and within a short period of time he was able to report a steady and welcome return of energy, together with a real improvement in all his other symptoms. One year later, he telephoned to say that he was very well: 'The discovery that I was hyperventilating was the turning point in my life.'

A simple breathing exercise for the anxious

Lie down on a bed in a quiet room away from all the pressures of the day, and loosen your belt and collar. Tighten all your muscle groups, one by one, and feel the relaxation flowing into each one as you release them. Start with your right hand, squeeze the fist really tight for a few seconds, and then relax it. Feel the relaxation flowing back into it, and take note of what it feels like to be relaxed. Now tighten the right arm muscles as tightly as you can for a few seconds, and relax. Repeat this for all the muscle groups, not forgetting your face, neck, shoulders, bottom and legs. This will only take a couple of minutes. Now place one hand on your upper chest and one hand on your abdomen, at the belt line. Breathe slowly through the nose into your abdomen. The hand on your chest should hardly move at all — if it does, you are breathing into the chest, not the abdomen. If at first you don't succeed, try again. You will get the hang of it, and when you do, begin to think in terms of rhythm: breathe in, count two, three; breathe out, two, three, and pause. Then breathe in again, count two, three; breathe out, two, three, and pause. You should be able to slow your breathing down to about six breaths per minute, but don't become a timekeeper! And don't hold your breath. Just concentrate on slowing down as much as you comfortably can, and stay there, in a relaxed state, for twenty minutes. Repeat the exercise twice a day until you feel better; thereafter once a day should suffice. This will correct your blood chemistry. The carbon dioxide level will come back to normal, and the respiratory centre will be bathed in this healthier chemical environment for as long as you stay there. As you repeat this simple exercise, the respiratory centre learns a new habit, just as it learned the bad habit originally. This time it will get used to a normal level of carbon dioxide in the blood and it will strive at all times to maintain it. Even when you are not consciously trying to breathe slowly, it will begin to control your breathing at this new and better pace. You will only breathe faster or deeper when exercise demands it. Even those who suffer from panic attacks can be taught how to control them, and hopefully prevent them altogether, by adopting this exercise. Whenever they feel the panic rising, they can simply control their breathing, slowing it down consciously, and thereby abort the attack before it ever really gets off the ground.

Case history

Anne is a 27-year-old teacher and mother of two active children. She complained of feeling tired all the time, and had done so for at least two years. In addition, she had nausea, loss of appetite, frequent loose bowel motions, headaches and pains in her chest. These made her feel a little short of breath. On a few occasions she had felt very panicky. During these episodes she experienced a worsening of symptoms, and in particular felt utterly exhausted. She could see that she was under considerable stress at work and at home with the demands of being a wife, mother and teacher. We discussed her situation at length. She was indeed going through a stressful patch, and she was obviously anxious as she spoke. She had never fully understood the cause of her symptoms (they had never been explained to her), and she had become quite worried about them: 'What if I have some serious condition?' The basis of her symptoms was explained in detail, and she was taught the simple breathing exercise (above) to carry out at home. One month later she reported a vast improvement in her energy and general well-being, with the disappearance of virtually all the symptoms. She remained just a little tired — but what working mother isn't?

Other treatment possibilities

The underlying anxiety disorder and/or phobia should be treated by an expert in the field. This sometimes involves medication, but it often involves cognitive behavioural therapy, in which graded exposures to the object or situation of fear may lead to the complete resolution of the phobia.

Why some non-anxious people become anxious and hyperventilate

Anxiety and panic feelings can be induced in healthy volunteers by infusing lactate into their bloodstream. Now that's interesting, isn't it? This is another example of a physical agent leading to a psychological reaction. So we have to say that anxiety, like depression, is not just all in the mind! Come back again to the thyroid gland. We saw that hypothyroidism may lead to depression. Now we consider the over-active gland: it may lead to anxiety. And this anxiety responds fully and dramatically to thyroid corrective treatment. So was this anxiety psychological or physical? Physical. Similarly, patients with life-threatening allergy (anaphylaxis) sometimes experience a feeling of impending doom as one of their first allergic (physical) symptoms.

Hysteria and Hypochondriasis

7

We come now to the last and least common psychiatric diagnosis given to the fatigued. See if you can spot the essential features in the following case history.

Case history

Gillian was in her forties before she first came to my clinic. She had faxed a summary of her complaints to my office before her appointment in the hope of making it easier to assess her. This was in the days of thermal fax paper that came out of the facsimile in one continuous roll. Her list was so long that I stood at one end of the corridor in my office and, holding one end of the paper, rolled the fax out like a red carpet to see how far it would stretch. Seventeen feet! Her symptoms were described in very distressing fashion, each one worse than the next. Some of the main headings included: chronic fatigue, burning eyes, swollen throat, pains in the ears, belching, mucus coming down from the sinuses, difficulty getting to sleep and difficulty waking up, chest pain, muscle pains, hives, palpitations, going hot and cold, sore lips, headaches, bloating abdomen, weakness, funny taste in the mouth, and on and on and on. There was also a list of all the other doctors she had been to see over the years, together with all the investigations and hospital admissions she had been through. Without exception, every single investigation was normal. Nor had there been any abnormality found on physical examination. When she turned up for her appointment, she added quite substantially to her faxed list, principally by enhancing the language used to describe her symptoms. Adjectives such as awful, terrible, excruciating and agonising were frequently invoked. Any attempt to explore her underlying emotions sent her into a flap and brought nothing but tearful accusations: 'You're just like all the others. You don't believe me.' As if to prove the point, she then swooned on to the floor, clutching her throat, coughing and spluttering and breathing noisily. She recovered from this distressing episode after a little gentle reassurance and encouragement. But ultimately we got nowhere. Gillian has what we used to call hysteria. Nowadays we call it somatisation. This condition is most common in females, affecting anywhere from 0.2 to 2 per cent of women at some point in their lives. Importantly, it always starts before they reach the age of 30.

There is no doubt at all that Gillian is suffering terribly, but what is really going on? In the first case, let us be absolutely clear about one thing. She is not deliberately inventing her symptoms — she has no voluntary control over them. If she had, we would call her a malingerer. She may be flamboyant and annoying in her presentation, but she is not a nasty person. She has severe psychological distress and this is being expressed in her body, or rather in bodily *sensations*, and in the way she presents these to the outside world. No medical explanation can ever be found for her symptoms, and she will usually refuse any psychological or psychiatric input. If the first doctor cannot 'sort out her problem' (and they never can, 'they're useless') she will go to another, and then another, and so on throughout her entire life. She will live just as long as anybody else, but she will spend ten times more than average on her health care.

Secondly, her symptoms are *not* psychosomatic. This is important, for there is much misunderstanding about this. A psychosomatic symptom is one in which a physical disorder is made worse by a psychological trigger. For example, a migraine headache triggered by stress would represent a psychosomatic phenomenon. We understand the mechanism of the headache: it is the physical (somatic) expression of a psychological (psycho) trigger. In hysteria there is no physical expression, no physical mechanism, no somatic component that can explain the symptom. We all have psychosomatic symptoms from time to time.

Thirdly, there may be some real gain in all of this for Gillian. After all, she's not doing it just for the fun of it. She is genuinely distressed, but what is the net effect of her illness experience? Does her husband have to drop everything and tend to her every need? Does she escape from some responsibility? Does she thrive on the attention she gets from doctors and nurses and friends? Does she feel unable to relate to society in any other way but through illness? We may never find out the answers to these questions; they are often too deeply buried.

We can be sure of this, however. There is a 90 per cent chance that she will be stuck like this for the next ten years. And if we meet her again at that stage, we could be saying the very same thing with the same conviction, i.e. there is a 90 per cent chance of her still being like this in a further ten years' time. Some of these patients are eventually diagnosed with a genuine disease, but that should come as no surprise: somatisation patients are not immortal!

We also need to say a word about the poor hypochondriac. On the face of it, he may be hard to distinguish from the somatiser. He too may have multiple unexplained symptoms, but there is a crucial difference. He is genuinely worried that he has a nasty disease which the doctors cannot find. Nor is he reassured by extensive investigation or multiple medical opinions.

Doctors must always be careful about making these diagnoses. There are many conditions that we cannot yet explain, including the symptom complex of chronic fatigue syndrome, to name but one, and we cannot dismiss these simply because we cannot explain them. Thus, to prematurely invoke the diagnosis of somatisation or hypochondriasis is always a dangerous mistake. However, if we stick to established diagnostic criteria, we will reduce our risk of error. The criteria for somatisation are summarised in the following table:

Do I have somatisation?

Tick if yes

1. A multitude of physical complaints experienced over several years, starting before the age of 30, and for which medical intervention was sought.	
2. Pain in at least four different sites: head, tummy, back, during intercourse etc.	
3. Gastrointestinal symptoms: including at least two of the following: nausea, vomiting, diarrhoea, bloating.	
4. Sexual symptoms: any symptom related to sex other than pain (disinterest, impotence, ejaculatory failure, excessive menstrual bleeding etc.)	
5. Nervous system symptoms: any symptom suggestive of a neurological disease such as paralysis, double vision, loss of balance etc.	
6. The symptoms cannot be explained medically.	
7. The symptoms are not deliberately feigned.	

If you have ticked *all* of the boxes above, then you probably have a somatisation disorder.

There are also incomplete forms of somatisation disorder. In these cases there may be a single debilitating symptom rather than the whole plethora of symptoms listed above. The symptom in question still defies medical explanation, i.e. there is still no physical component involved. These are called somatoform or conversion disorders, so called because the symptom is seen to be the 'conversion' of psychological conflict into bodily sensations. In classical cases, conversion symptoms achieve two things for the patient: the immediate relief of their psychological distress and the secondary 'benefits' of being ill, such as postponing important decisions, avoiding responsibility, or getting loved ones to dance attendance. I mention this here because one of the most common conversion symptoms encountered in practice is fatigue (it used to be paralysis). There have been occasional case reports in the medical literature in which patients with 'chronic fatigue syndrome' have improved once their internal psychological conflicts have been addressed. For example, a young girl who had suppressed rage directed against her mother started to 'recover her energy' once this issue was explored with a skilled psychologist. To my mind, she did not have a true chronic fatigue syndrome (that's why I used quotes); she had a conversion disorder:

- Her rage was converted to fatigue and inactivity — psychologists call this 'passive aggression'.
- Her primary gain was the immediate relief of her psychological conflict ('How do I deal with this anger?')
- The secondary gain was getting her mother worried about her and tending to her every need.
- Her recovery was facilitated by helping her find a different and healthier mode of expression.

If you suspect that you have somatisation or a related disorder, you will need courage to explore this possibility at greater depth. You will also need expert help to find a new approach to expressing and resolving your very real psychological distress.

8 Fatigue as a Symptom of Physical Disease

We move on now to consider fatigue in the context of physical disease. This will provide us with a sense of continuity, for we are still following our original one hundred hypothetical patients. We have dealt with the psychological and psychiatric disorders; now we look at the 5 per cent who are eventually given physical explanations for their fatigue.

We are still particularly interested in patients who present themselves to a doctor because they are feeling tired all the time. This is their specific reason for attendance. They may admit to other symptoms when questioned, but they consider these to be less important. A patient who feels truly fatigued will often say, 'Relieve me of my tiredness. I can cope with the rest.'

A typical family doctor can expect to see anywhere from one to five such patients in every one hundred consultations. Admittedly, this figure varies a bit across different nations. For example, doctors in Canada or France might see six or seven cases in the same time frame. We are not sure why this apparent difference exists, but it may have to do with the way different cultures express their illness (rather than reflect a true difference in the incidence of fatigue).

In any case, this is an interesting scenario and one that lends itself to another survey. This time we could sit outside the doctor's office and interview every patient as they leave the consulting room. If we ask them why they consulted in the first place, we would, of course, come up with the same one to 7 per cent who attend primarily because they are tired. But we would also discover that 16 per cent of males and 30 per cent of females who attend for *other* reasons would also admit to tiredness. And if we conducted a similar survey in a hospital setting, we would find the very same thing. Fatigue is the single most common symptom experienced by those who are ill.

As a symptom, then, fatigue does not give us any clues as to its cause. It is far too non-specific and it can accompany virtually any physical or mental illness. However, it is reassuring to note that only 5 per cent of the fatigued are suffering from a known physical disease, although not all would agree with me there. Some of my worst-affected chronic fatigue patients will sit in despair on the verge of tears and tell me that they would rather be diagnosed with cancer than have to live with unexplained fatigue: 'At least I'd know why I was so tired', they'd say. This is not a death wish; it's desperation. They are driven to distraction by the uncertainty of it all. We will come back to this problem later on. Meanwhile, let us take a closer look at the most common physical explanations of fatigue. These are (i) a low blood count and (ii) disorders of the thyroid gland. Mention will also be made of miscellaneous physical conditions that can sometimes present as profound fatigue.

Anaemia — low blood count

Blood is made up of two components, cells and plasma. The main cells found in blood are either white or red. The white cells have a major function in immunity: they protect us from infection and they mop up other cells that threaten to turn cancerous. The major function of red cells is to transport oxygen around the body. The oxygen-carrying capacity of red cells is determined by their haemoglobin content. When we speak of a low blood count, we are referring specifically to a low haemoglobin, and to the associated changes in the size and shape of the red cells that carry it — the correct term is anaemia. As you would expect, the main symptoms are fatigue and poor physical performance. Other symptoms occur, but these depend to a large extent on the cause of the anaemia. Anaemia most commonly results from the impaired manufacture of haemoglobin. Iron, vitamin B12, folate, protein, vitamin C and copper are all required for the adequate production of haemoglobin, so a deficiency of any of these will lead to the problem. The manufacture of blood cells may also be impaired by disease, such as arthritis or a hormonal problem. The other main cause of anaemia is blood loss. Women are especially at risk because of their monthly menstrual loss, but parasites can also cause excessive loss in both men and women.

Iron deficiency anaemia

Iron deficiency is the most common nutritional deficiency worldwide, affecting up to 50 per cent of the population in certain parts of Africa and Asia, and some 5 to 15 per cent of the North American and European populations. The people most at risk of iron deficiency include the following:

- infants and toddlers (aged 6 months–2½ years) of whom 24 per cent have an inadequate dietary intake.
- young children (under 4) of whom 84 per cent have an inadequate dietary intake.
- adolescents, particularly those who become pregnant, or who diet to get thin.
- fertile women whose iron loss with each menstrual cycle may prove difficult to replenish, and in whom the demands of pregnancy on iron stores are great.
- the elderly, among whom 6 per cent of men and 12 per cent of women are deficient.
- vegetarians and vegans, with particular risk to those of Indian origin.
- socially and economically deprived individuals.

The consequences of iron deficiency are considerable, and include fatigue, poor physical and work performance, anaemia, and behavioural problems in childhood. There is also an adverse effect on immune function leading to more frequent infections.

The matter of iron deficiency is more complex than may at first appear. It's not just a question of making sure you have enough iron on your plate; you need to know what happens to the iron once you've swallowed it. For example, a third of fertile women have an iron intake well below the recommended level, and a third have signs of iron deficiency, but they are not the same thirds! In other words, many women with a low intake do not develop iron deficiency, and many with iron deficiency have a (supposedly) adequate intake (the same has been found in children). This suggests that the *efficiency* of iron absorption is just as important as an adequate dietary intake. It is not good enough to say, 'I have a healthy diet.' We must make sure that you are absorbing it properly as well.

The absorption of iron from the gut into the bloodstream is probably genetically determined: we are either efficient or inefficient absorbers. Furthermore, the absorption of iron from any given meal may vary from less than one per cent to more than 50 per cent! There are two reasons for this. Firstly, there are two forms of iron — haem and non-haem. As the name suggests, iron that is already part of a haemoglobin molecule is called haem iron; iron that is not attached to anything is called non-haem iron. Foods which contain haemoglobin (meat, fish, poultry, and their products) are therefore rich sources of haem iron. Dairy products and plant foods contain non-haem iron. This is important because haem iron is absorbed three times more readily than non-haem iron. Secondly, animal proteins interact with the human intestine to further enhance iron absorption. Vitamin C has a similar enhancing effect. Therefore, meals which contain haem iron and vitamin C (e.g. fruit or fruit juice) offer the best in terms of iron absorption. Conversely, iron absorption is inhibited by bran and phytic acids (which occur naturally in whole cereals), by calcium (in milk) and by polyphenols (in tea and vegetables). In the light of this, it is easy to see how a vegetarian diet predisposes a patient to iron deficiency.

The dangers of excessive iron

It might be tempting, but it would be quite wrong to start filling ourselves up with iron in the hope of getting more energy. Too much iron can be dangerous.

Excess iron:

- has a propensity to favour neoplastic growth, and there is some evidence of an association between excess iron and cancer.
- may be a risk factor in heart disease.

- may be implicated in sudden infant death.
- may be a risk factor in toxaemia in pregnancy.
- leads to the deposition of iron in various organs in patients with a condition called haemochromatosis.

Vitamin B12 and folate deficiencies (pernicious anaemia)

Vitamin B12 deficiency leads to abnormalities in the blood, small intestine and the nervous system. Signs and symptoms include fatigue, anaemia, glossitis (inflamed tongue), malabsorption of other nutrients, pins and needles, weakness, and eventually a degeneration of the spinal cord. The latter is serious, leading to a form of paralysis, and is not easily corrected even when subsequently treated with B12 supplements. This is why the associated anaemia was christened 'pernicious' — it's not just a low blood count.

Vitamin B12 is also needed for folate to work properly. Thus B12 deficiency leads to what we call a functional folate deficiency. In other words, there may be plenty of folate about, but it just won't function in the absence of B12. However, folate deficiency arising in the presence of B12 will still cause anaemia and fatigue.

Normal vitamin B12 levels depend on (i) an adequate dietary intake, (ii) adequate digestion, and (iii) adequate absorption. Although dietary deficiency is rare, many elderly people, especially those who live on their own, or who have difficulty obtaining and preparing food, are at risk of poor intake. Once ingested, the vitamin must then be released from the protein to which it is bound. Free B12 is then absorbed into the bloodstream, but only with the help of a transport molecule called intrinsic factor, which is manufactured in the stomach. Many conditions affecting the stomach may therefore lead to B12 deficiency, even if there is an adequate dietary intake. Thus, insufficient acid in the stomach (hypochlorhydria), degeneration of the lining of the stomach (atrophic gastritis) and/or gastric infection will all lead to deficiency. Once again the elderly are particularly vulnerable in this regard. Furthermore, sometimes the immune system gets it wrong and produces antibodies to intrinsic factor or to the cells that produce it, leading to problems with absorption. And as if that wasn't enough, those who have to take a daily dose of aspirin (to prevent heart disease or stroke) may find that it also interferes with B12 absorption. The treatment of B12 deficiency anaemia takes the absorption problem into consideration — B12 is given by injection, thus avoiding the gut entirely. Strict vegans develop pernicious anaemia over several years. It takes a while because we are equipped with a very efficient recycling mechanism for B12 — we hang on to it and use it again and again.

All B12 in nature is made by bugs and eventually finds its way into the food chain. Plants do not contain any B12, except when they are contaminated by microbes. Most of our B12 therefore comes from meat and meat products, fish and shellfish, poultry and eggs, with lesser amounts in milk. Some forms of seaweed contain microbial B12 and would be acceptable to both vegans and vegetarians.

Folate is found in foliage, hence the name. Thus green leafy vegetables are one of the best sources, but it is also found in liver, kidney, nuts and wholegrain cereals.

The diagnosis of anaemia

A simple blood test will show whether you are anaemic. The haemoglobin concentration can easily be measured in the laboratory. The size and shape of the red cells will also give clues as to the cause of the anaemia. For example, small pale red cells indicate iron deficiency anaemia, whereas fat cells suggest B12 or folate deficiency. Iron, B12 and folate levels can also be measured separately. This is useful because brain symptoms such as fatigue and depression can sometimes precede the anaemia in cases of early or borderline deficiency.

Disorders of the thyroid gland

The thyroid gland is located in front of the voice box (larynx) in the neck. It produces thyroid hormones. We do not know exactly how these exert their influence, but we do know that they speed up metabolism throughout the body. They are particularly important in childhood for normal growth, for mental development and for a successful passage through puberty. In adult life they are essential for regulating metabolism. This includes the metabolism of the brain, the heart and the intestinal tract etc.

The main thyroid hormones are thyroxine (which we abbreviate to T4) and tri-iodothyronine (which we abbreviate to T3). T4 is converted to T3 outside the thyroid gland by a series of enzymes. This is an important step because T3 is far more active than T4. As you can tell by the name (iodo-), iodine is an important constituent of the thyroid hormones. Inadequate supplies of iodine in the diet will lead to a functional thyroid deficiency, and iodine replacement restores full thyroid function. The thyroid gland actively takes up iodine from the bloodstream, and responds to low iodine levels by increasing its size, giving the classical goitre — a thyroid swelling in the neck. Iodine deficiency is rare nowadays, except in areas where the soil content of iodine is depleted. The addition of iodine to table salt in many countries has gone a long way to eradicating this problem.

In health, the thyroid gland is regulated by the brain, and this is how it 'knows' how much hormone to produce. Specifically, the pituitary gland secretes a hormone called thyroid stimulating hormone (TSH). TSH travels in the blood to the thyroid gland and provides the correct amount of 'stimulation', and hence the correct amount of T4 and T3 are produced. To complicate matters further, the pituitary is also regulated! It will release TSH only when it is 'told' to do so by another hormone (TSH-releasing hormone) which is produced in the hypothalamus (see Figure 1). Finally, there is a feedback loop from the body to the brain which lets the brain know whether there is enough thyroid hormone around or not. If there is sufficient, the level of TSH drops back a bit; if there is a lack, the TSH level moves up a notch. I know this is all very technical, but the main point is simple: the thyroid gland is regulated by a very sophisticated system in the brain. The importance of this will become clear shortly.

Meanwhile, let us come back to our principal concern, namely, the relationship between thyroid disorders and fatigue. The thyroid may become underactive (hypothyroid) or over-active (hyperthyroid), and both may cause fatigue. We would expect anything which lowers our metabolism to result in fatigue, and so we are not unduly surprised to learn that hypothyroidism quickly leads to a loss of energy; but hyperthyroidism is also exhausting.

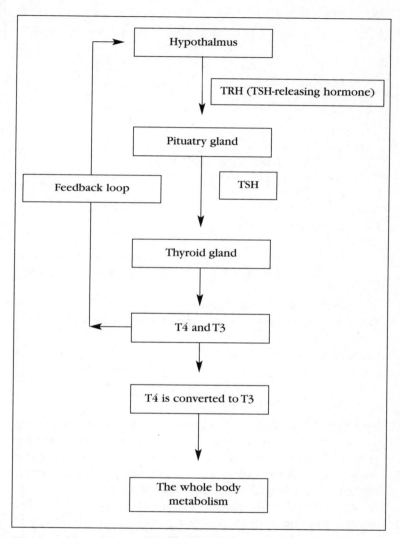

Figure 1. The control of thyroid function

Hypothyroidism

The symptom complex of hypothyroidism is as follows:

1. gradual slowing of general metabolism, leading to
2. mental sluggishness
3. depression
4. fatigue
5. weight gain
6. intolerance of cold
7. sluggish bowel function (constipation)
8. sluggish heart rate (slower heart rate)
9. sluggish reflexes
10. dry skin
11. menstrual irregularities
12. hair loss
13. hoarse voice, and other alterations in voice (particularly noticeable in singers who can no longer reach the higher notes)
14. puffiness of the face and legs (myxoedema)
15. and in extreme cases, hypothermia (falling body temperature) and coma.
16. There is also a rare form of mental illness associated with severe hypothyroidism called myxoedema madness.

CAUSES OF HYPOTHYROIDISM

Hypothyroidism may result from the disruption to any part of the pathway from the hypothalamus to the thyroid gland itself. Most cases are idiopathic (we don't know the cause) failures of the thyroid gland itself; others are caused by the auto-immune destruction of thyroid cells (in which the immune system 'attacks' the thyroid gland in the mistaken belief that it is 'foreign' rather than 'self'). In rare cases the problem has to do with the failure of the stimulating system to work effectively.

Hyperthyroidism

As you would expect, the symptoms of hyperthyroidism are almost the opposite to those of hypothyroidism. But as we have already said, fatigue may also be a prominent symptom here:

1. gradual speeding up of the metabolism, leading to
2. mental overactivity, restlessness or anxiety and other emotional symptoms
3. tremor (the shakes), especially in the hands
4. fatigue
5. weight loss
6. intolerance of heat
7. over-active bowel function (diarrhoea)
8. over-active heart rate (faster heart rate and sometimes palpitations)
9. very brisk reflexes
10. excessive sweating, and
11. in some cases the eyes protrude, giving a staring appearance (exophthalmos).

CAUSES OF HYPERTHYROIDISM

Hyperthyroidism most commonly results from an auto-immune disease (Graves' disease). It may also result from single or multiple nodules in the thyroid. These are rogue cells which spew out thyroid hormone without respect to the regulating influence of the pituitary.

The diagnosis of thyroid disease

There are several laboratory tests which assess thyroid function. For example, we can measure T4, and we can reasonably assume that T4 levels will be lower than normal in hypothyroidism and higher than normal in hyperthyroidism. This is generally true in clinical practice. However, as in all biological systems, there is a range of normal levels. Thus a level of 60 nmol per litre of blood would be normal for some people, but others might need 160 nmol. That's quite a range. So if we measured *your* T4 and found that it was 80 nmol/l, how would we know that this was a normal level for *you*? We wouldn't! To get around this problem, we can ask your brain what it thinks! And, specifically, we can ask your pituitary gland. If your TSH level is normal, then we can assume that 80 nmol/l of T4 is sufficient for you. If, on the other hand, your TSH level is elevated, we can safely assume that 80 nmol/l is not sufficient for you. Your brain is sending out more TSH in an attempt to get the thyroid to produce more T4.

The thyroid tests may be affected by medicines, pregnancy, other illnesses, following surgery, and/or in nutritional disturbances. But, apart from these isolated cases, they are reliable. In fact the TSH level is thought to be so reliable that many laboratories use it alone to screen for thyroid function. A normal TSH is said to invariably mean normal thyroid function. In hypothyroidism the TSH level can reach for the sky; in hyperthyroidism it may be undetectable. The treatment of thyroid disorders is said to be successful when the TSH and T4 levels come back within the normal range.

The argument

However, there may be more to this story than meets the eye. Some doctors, for example, have noted that the relationship between thyroid symptoms and thyroid hormone levels is not as clear or consistent as outlined above, particularly in relation to hypothyroidism. They claim that a patient should be treated for an underactive thyroid if they have the *symptoms* of hypothyroidism, irrespective of the biochemical test. In effect, they are saying 'treat the patient — not the blood test', and they are calling for more research in this area. So far, they have published a few studies in which patients with normal blood tests but clinical symptoms of hypothyroidism have improved significantly on thyroid hormone treatment. In fact, some of these patients had been previously investigated and given a diagnosis of chronic fatigue syndrome — and that's why I'm spending so much time on this subject. Perhaps we have been missing cases of clinical hypothyroidism by relying too much on laboratory tests. In support of their theory, they have produced research findings which suggest that TSH and T4 estimates are poor indicators of thyroid status, and they have also proposed more accurate tests, but these are not widely available as yet. Meanwhile, there is a strong case for judging each individual patient on clinical grounds in relation to thyroid function. Patients with clinical hypothyroidism but normal thyroid blood tests have been found to have the following symptoms:

Fatigue as a Symptom of Physical Disease

Yes =1 No = 0

1. chronic fatigue	
2. depression	
3. intolerance to cold	
4. headache	
5. poor memory or concentration	
6. muscle cramps	
7. constipation	
8. joint pains	
9. changes in appearance	
10. changes in skin or hair	
11. reduced libido	
12. puffy face or extremities	
13. blurring of vision	
14. slow heart rate	
15. difficulty swallowing	
16. enlarged tongue	
17. swollen thyroid gland	
18. increased weight	
19. a slow ankle reflex (tested by the doctor)	
Total score	/19

The higher your score, the more likely it is that you have an underactive thyroid.

This is a composite list of symptoms taken from published studies on clinical hypothyroidism (in the presence of normal blood tests). These symptoms disappeared in 76 per cent of patients studied, and a further 17 per cent of patients improved significantly. That represents an overall response rate of 93 per cent, which is strong evidence that these symptoms were related to hypothyroidism in the first place, in spite of the normal laboratory tests.

I'm sure you will appreciate that this is a very controversial approach to thyroid disorders, but hopefully the issues raised will be addressed by future research. The important thing for us to remember is that some patients with profound fatigue, and who would otherwise be considered as cases of chronic fatigue syndrome, improve dramatically when treated with thyroid hormone.

Miscellany

It has already been stated that fatigue is a non-specific symptom that may accompany virtually any illness. But some diseases are noted for the degree of fatigue they cause. Diseases of the nervous system are foremost among these. Multiple sclerosis, for example, frequently causes debilitating fatigue. But in this and similar cases other signs and symptoms of the underlying disease will usually be present. I say usually because sometimes the fatigue precedes the manifestations of the underlying illness by several months. Remember that we are now talking of a *tiny* minority of patients.

These diseases are mentioned here for the sake of completeness, and not to instil terror. In the last ten years of practice I have assessed thousands of patients with fatigue, and I can assure you that the chances of discovering some nasty underlying disease are very remote.

It is also salutary to note the case reports of mistaken diagnoses that appear from time to time in the medical literature. We would be particularly interested in patients who were diagnosed as suffering from chronic fatigue syndrome and who were later found to have some other explanation for their fatigue. Chronic sinusitis, rare forms of rheumatism, sleep disorders, parasites, rare endocrine tumours, poisoning and low phosphate levels have all been mistaken for chronic fatigue syndrome. Finally, we must not forget that patients with chronic fatigue syndrome are not immune from other completely unrelated diseases.

Case history

Andrew was a 50-year-old prison officer who got an acute infection in his middle ear (labarynthitis) three years ago. He had been unable to work since then. He had a clear case of postviral fatigue syndrome, and was responding rather slowly to treatment. Initial investigations were all normal, so we proceeded to manage his case in the usual way. Because of his slow progress, he had repeated investigations which were again normal, including a thyroid test. Some months later he was called for a medical by his employer. On this occasion his TSH was sky high, prompting excited phone calls around the country between one doctor and another. I could hear a rather agitated voice coming down the line at me: 'This man is extremely hypothyroid, dangerously so! He never had ME. In fact ME doesn't exist. He was hypothyroid all along.' I tried to point out that his TSH was perfectly normal only ninety days before, but I wasn't getting through. Then Andrew phoned me: 'What do you think?' he asked. 'They think that I'm hypothyroid and you're an eejit', he said, laughing. Andrew knew that his TSH was perfect when he was at his worst, and he strongly suspected that this was a red herring. It was. After adequate treatment with thyroid hormone his TSH returned to normal, but he felt no difference at all. He was still debilitated by fatigue. We laughed again at the whole débâcle and continued to manage his CFS in the usual way.

It is good medical practice to keep an open mind when dealing with fatigue states. This involves taking a fresh look at the case every six to twelve months, particularly if little or no progress is being made, or if some new symptom or sign appears. If progress is being made, there is no need for endless tests. The evaluation and management of chronic fatigue states is outlined in Section 4.

Section 3

Forgotten Causes of Fatigue

(I) FATIGUE AND SLEEP

Chapter 9 Normal Sleep Pattern and Sleep Requirements

Chapter 10 Chronic Sleep Deprivation

Chapter 11 Sleep Disorders

(II) FATIGUE AND DIET

Chapter 12 Diet, Mood and Energy

Chapter 13 Overweight and Obesity

Chapter 14 Nutritional Deficiency

Chapter 15 Food Allergy and Intolerance

Chapter 16 Caffeine

Chapter 17 Hypoglycaemia — Low Blood Sugar

(III) FATIGUE AND GERMS

Chapter 18 The Truth about Candida

Chapter 19 Parasites, Bacteria and Viruses

(IV) FATIGUE AND CHEMICALS

Chapter 20 Multiple Chemical Sensitivity Syndrome

Normal Sleep Pattern and Sleep Requirements

9

Sleep is a fundamental biological requirement as important to health as food and water. By its regular provision we are maintained in a state of physical and mental well-being. It is the means whereby healthy individuals dispose of tiredness and 'recharge their batteries'. It is obvious that any disruption to this process, particularly if protracted, will inevitably result in a state of fatigue. In spite of this, many continue — willingly or unwillingly — to deprive themselves of its ministry. People who suffer from a specific sleep disorder will also suffer profound disruptions to their quality of life. A description of normal sleep, and of the consequences of insufficient or disordered sleep, will help to emphasise the importance of sleep to health in general, and fatigue in particular.

Normal sleep pattern

Sleep remains a mystery with unfathomable secrets. In spite of intensive research, we still know very little about it. What we can say for sure, however, is that sleep is not a passive state. The brain never really switches off at all. If it did, we would die! There is a complex arrangement of what we might call 'shift work': those brain cells which were active during the day shift are allowed to wind down for the night; another set, quiet during the day, takes over the night shift. It is the study of the electrical activity of these cells which has provided us with most of our present understanding. The electrical waves which they generate can be recorded on a graph, the electro-encephalogram (*encephalo* meaning brain) or EEG for short. While sleep may feel like a uniform state to us (apart perhaps from the occasional dream), it never is. EEG studies reveal that it consists of five distinct stages. Of course, as far as we are concerned, we simply fall asleep in blissful ignorance of the complex goings on in the brain.

The familiar feeling of increasing drowsiness which precedes sleep is due to the gradual build-up of neurotransmitters (chemical substances) in the brain. This heralds the conclusion of the day shift and, as the night shift cells take over, we drift imperceptibly into the first stage of sleep. Brain activity now diminishes rapidly. Within forty-five to sixty minutes, we will have plunged through the second and third stages, to the fourth and deepest stage of sleep. The waves seen on the EEG throughout this time become progressively slower, reflecting the brain's relative inactivity. Hence, these stages are known collectively as slow wave (SW) sleep. It is difficult to waken out of SW sleep.

Brain activity now increases again, returning right through the first stage, and beyond it, into a fifth stage. Peculiar to the fifth stage is the unmistakable rapid movement of the eyes behind closed lids, from which it derives the name 'rapid eye movement' (REM) sleep. If we wake at this time (and we are more likely to do so) we will, most probably, report the vivid dreams for which this stage is renowned. In contrast, subjects woken out of SW sleep seldom report dreaming. What they remember is a vague sense of having had 'thoughts on their minds'. The almost universal experience of not being able to sleep well during times of stress can be explained on the basis of anxious thought intruding on SW sleep.

The first period of REM sleep continues for five to ten minutes before the brain slows once again in pursuit of the deeper stages, and thus the whole cycle is repeated, at regular intervals, throughout the night. In later cycles, stages 3 and 4 are abandoned, more time is spent in stages 1 and 2, and the episodes of REM sleep become longer. In all, 75 per cent of sleep is spent in SW sleep, and 25 per cent in REM sleep (see Diagram 1).

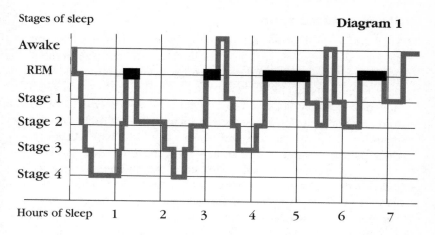

Stages of sleep **Diagram 1**

The brain retains overall command of body function throughout sleep. It does so by controlling the release of numerous hormones. These travel through the blood to distant organs, where they exert profound effects. On one hand, the stress hormones (adrenaline and cortisol) fall to their lowest levels. This results in a fall in pulse rate, blood pressure and blood sugar. Consequently, body temperature cools, oxygen consumption declines and metabolism is reduced by about 20 per cent. On the other hand, hormones which facilitate tissue repair rise to their highest levels. These include growth hormone, prolactin and testosterone. The reverse occurs during waking hours. Virtually every hormone and neurotransmitter in the body demonstrates this same pattern of peaks and troughs over a twenty-four hour period. This is called the 'circadian rhythm' (from the Latin *circa diem*, meaning about a day). The sleep/wake cycle is the bedrock upon which the circadian rhythm is founded, and our general health depends very much on its balanced harmony.

The usual experience of healthy people is that they wake in the morning feeling refreshed. It may take them thirty minutes or so to become fully alert, but chemical balance has been restored to their brains, and their bodies have enjoyed prolonged periods of rest and repair. This is restorative sleep, and it should be common to all.

Sleep requirements

Most adults need seven to nine hours' sleep each night. Thus, on average, we spend one third of our lives in bed. This requirement changes with age: typically, newborn babes need sixteen hours a day; 5-year olds twelve hours; 10-year olds ten hours; teenagers nine hours; and adults seven to nine hours. The elderly, because of frequent wakeful periods, sleep significantly less at night, but the majority make up the loss during the day with naps. Although their pattern changes, their total sleep time does not. There is, however, enormous variation in sleep requirements between individuals. A few, for some unknown reason, can function quite happily on very little sleep. With paltry amounts, they can work energetically, concentrate their minds with ease and enjoy an action-packed social life. They complain of neither insomnia nor fatigue. Others may not be able to function unless they get a regular ten hours or more, but if they do get it, they can work like Trojans and cheerfully accomplish a great deal during their waking hours. They have no complaint to make about their health. If you wake refreshed and feel well during the day, you are clearly getting enough good quality sleep, be it five hours or ten.

By way of illustration, consider the US Army general, George Custer. He required eight hours' sleep every night, except during his campaigns when his requirement rose to nine hours. Nobody would have called him lazy! In contrast, the great preacher Charles Wesley made a point of getting out of bed at 4 a.m. each morning. He spent a few hours in prayer and Bible reading, and then went for a brisk walk before sitting down to breakfast at 8 a.m. During his lifetime he covered some 250,000 miles. He must have been one of the most widely travelled men of his day, and most of it was on horseback — an amazing achievement for any man, let alone on so little sleep.

How much sleep do I need?

Given what we have just said about individual differences in sleep requirements, how can you be sure of your own sleep requirements? The best way to answer this question is to take a 'sleeping holiday'! This does not mean that you sleep around the clock; in fact, daytime naps are specifically discouraged. What it does mean is that sleep is given priority over every other activity. It is the main purpose of the holiday.

For the first few evenings, go to bed when you are feeling sleepy, not before, but certainly not too long after the onset of drowsiness. Initially, you may feel sleepy earlier in the evening than you would like, but go with it, even if it means that you miss out on other activities. Don't commit yourself to anything that would require an early start the next day. Rather, sleep until your eyes open. You will catch up on your sleep debt within a few days (although it may take up to six weeks to fully recover from severe sleep deprivation). Your sleep pattern will find its own rhythm. You will start to get sleepy at approximately the same time each evening and you will sleep for approximately the same length of time each night. This is your basic sleep requirement. Bear in mind that this requirement may increase during times of illness or stress, but it will never decrease. You may manage fairly well on less sleep for short periods, but you will always need to catch up on lost sleep before it catches up on you.

By way of example, let us suppose that your sleep requirement turns out to be eight hours per night. That's fine on holidays, you may say, but what happens when you get back to the real world? The pressures of life may demand that you get out of bed at 7 a.m. or earlier, and may prevent you from getting to bed before midnight. So now you are getting seven hours' sleep per night instead of eight. Does it really matter? Yes, it does. Think of it like this: seven hours' sleep per night, seven nights a week, gives you a total of forty-nine hours' sleep per week. But you need eight hours' sleep, seven nights a week, a total sleep requirement of fifty-six hours. This represents a sleep debt of seven hours per week. In other words, it's the equivalent of missing one full night's sleep every week!

The influence of food intolerance on sleep requirement

Some patients report a change in their sleep requirement when, in the pursuit of relief from some other apparently unrelated condition, they avoid foods to which they are found to be intolerant. Susan is one such person. She is a 45-year-old hotelier, who presented with a complaint of pressure pains on both sides of her head. She had a muzzy feeling and poor concentration. In addition, she felt nauseated almost every day. She had been admitted to hospital for investigation, but no explanation for her symptoms was forthcoming. She went to bed regularly at 11 p.m. and slept till 8 a.m. She ate a healthy diet, but admitted to a craving for sweet things. Indeed, she could not get herself going in the morning until she had eaten some form of sugar. After two weeks on a low allergy diet, her head cleared completely and the nausea ceased. Upon subsequent food challenges, she reacted strongly to milk, which she had half-suspected, and to white sugar, which she had not suspected at all. They both induced a feeling of heightened anxiety, poor concentration and muzzy headedness. As long as she avoids these foods she remains well. 'I wake at 6 a.m. every morning now. Is that all right?' She was surprised at the change. She felt great on rising and had taken to long walks before breakfast. She does not tire later in the day. Dealing with underlying food intolerance had unexpectedly changed her sleep requirement, and she felt the better for it. The interesting point here is that she appeared to be getting enough sleep, but it was of poor quality.

How do I know if I'm getting good quality sleep?

Before we answer this question, we need to make an important distinction between two related but quite different symptoms. We need to distinguish between the feelings of sleepiness and fatigue — they are not the same thing. Sleepiness brings with it a desire to sleep, sometimes an irresistible desire, and it is relieved by sleep. It is not just a feeling of tiredness. Fatigue, on the other hand, is quite different. It may have nothing whatever to do with a desire for sleep. It is more like a weakness, a lack of energy, or lethargy. Indeed, the fatigue that we are particularly interested in, the feeling of being tired all the time, is seldom relieved by sleep, unless, of course, it is associated with insufficient sleep! It is quite possible to experience both symptoms together; but it is equally possible to be *either* excessively tired *or* sleepy. So what about you? Are you tired, or sleepy, or both?

The Excessive Daytime Sleepiness questionnaire will help you sort this out. You simply rate your likelihood of falling asleep in various situations. The ratings are on a four point scale, with 0 representing a 'no chance' and 3 representing a 'high chance' of falling asleep. This may seem simplistic, but it has been shown by clinical trial to have the ability to distinguish between those who have a sleep disorder and those who do not. In other words, it is a reliable assessment of excessive daytime sleepiness. Take a few minutes to fill out the questionnaire. In doing so, keep in mind that we are referring to your usual routine of recent weeks and months. Some of the situations may not apply directly to you. In these cases give your 'best guess' answer. Add up your score, and compare it to the scores presented in the following Table. Don't worry about the big names — they will be explained shortly.

Excessive Daytime Sleepiness Questionnaire

Situations	Chance of dozing
Sitting and reading	
Watching TV	
Sitting inactive in a public place (e.g. a theatre or a meeting)	
As a passenger in a car for an hour without a break	
Lying down to rest in the afternoon when circumstances permit	
Sitting and talking to someone	
Sitting quietly after a lunch without alcohol	
In a car, while stopped for a few minutes in traffic	
Total	/24

Scoring scale:

0 = would never doze   1 = slight chance of dozing

2 = moderate chance of dozing   3 = high chance of dozing

Table 2. Excessive daytime sleepiness scores and associated
sleep disorders

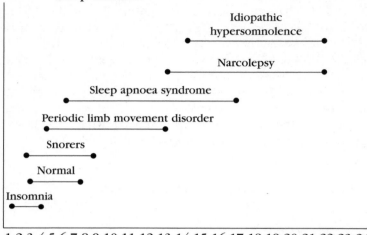

We can learn several things from this table. In the first place,
scores above 9–10 are always abnormal. They are an indication of
excessive daytime sleepiness, not just fatigue. Excessive daytime
sleepiness is almost always caused by insufficient or disordered
sleep. Common disorders include:

1. Chronic sleep deprivation (not included in the table).
2. Restless legs and periodic limb movement disorder (PLMD).
3. Sleep apnoea syndrome.
4. Narcolepsy.
5. Idiopathic hypersomnolence.

You will have noticed that there is some overlap between the
various sleep disorder scores, and between normal and abnormal
scores; and furthermore, that scores below 10 may or may not be
an indication of disordered sleep. In the latter cases, other
symptoms from the history would be taken into account in
formulating a diagnosis. Thus, milder cases of sleep apnoea and
PLMD may not experience excessive daytime sleepiness, but they
will have other symptoms (see below). Notice also that snoring

per se does not necessarily result in daytime sleepiness; it only becomes a problem when it is associated with sleep apnoea. Having said that, it may be a significant problem for the other people in the bedroom! Finally, insomnia is associated with fatigue, but it does not result in excessive daytime sleepiness. In fact, insomniacs have trouble falling asleep day *and* night; consequently they report decreased daytime sleepiness. Let us now examine sleep deprivation and sleep disorders in some detail.

Chronic Sleep Deprivation

As a society we have reduced our sleeping time by 20 per cent in the past one hundred years. We have also increased our work and travel load by an average of one full month per year. The result is that we now have an epidemic of sleep deprivation, with 65 per cent of adults admitting they don't get enough sleep. We are trying to achieve more and more on less and less sleep.

Case history

Eugene is a fairly typical example of this modern mania. He is a solicitor in his early fifties, whose wife persuaded him to attend my clinic. She was concerned about his increasing fatigue. He had no other symptoms of ill health, apart from elevated blood pressure. It turns out that his normal day starts at 6 a.m. with the unmerciful intrusion of an alarm clock across his unfinished sleep. He is forced into another day with body and brain still trying to process yesterday's burdens. After a few cups of coffee, he drives for ninety minutes through the commuter traffic to reach his office. He spends the day in the city, about his business, and then turns around again for the journey home. He finally sits down to a meal at 9 p.m. and collapses into bed at midnight. He knows it won't be long before he hears the dreaded bell again. Clearly, to search for another cause of fatigue would be a futile exercise — Eugene needs to sleep!

Sleep deprivation is not a trivial thing. In fact, it has such a devastating effect on body and soul that it has been used in brainwashing and torture regimes. Prisoners will start to hallucinate and their minds will fill with paranoid ideation within three days of total sleep deprivation. In other words, they go stark raving mad! Fortunately, this form of deprivation is rare. Much more common, and a bit more subtle, are the effects of partial sleep deprivation. It may seem obvious, but the consequences of not getting our full quota of sleep are enormous. For example, healthy volunteers, within one day of partial sleep deprivation, show a deterioration of both concentration and task performance. Further deprivation renders them incapable of coherent thought and unreliable in decision-making. This is followed by increased irritability, heightened anxiety and depressed mood. Needless to say, subjects in these studies complain of extreme fatigue. They are likely to fall asleep involuntarily, unless kept awake by a vigilant observer. The more chronic the sleep deprivation, the more numerous and troublesome are the associated symptoms. These are summarised in the following table.

Table 3. The symptoms of chronic sleep deprivation

	Yes = 1 No = 0
1. Fatigue	
2. Poor concentration and memory	
3. Poor task performance	
4. Difficulties with complex thought	
5. Unreliable decision-making	
6. Excessive daytime sleepiness	
7. Accidental sleep episodes	
8. Irritability, anxiety, depressed mood	
9. Stomach problems (indigestion and heartburn)	
10. Menstrual irregularities	
11. High blood pressure	
12. Weight gain	
13. Frequent infections	
14. Muscle pains	
(Those who are prone to migraine or epilepsy are more likely to suffer attacks when sleep deprived.)	
Total score	/14

Some of us, through force of habit, choose to stay up till the early hours of the morning. We have it in our power to control the amount of sleep we get. As such, we deserve little sympathy when we complain of fatigue, as we invariably do. But others, through pressure of work or other circumstances, have little choice but to forgo sleep. These have a more difficult problem.

Parental sleep deprivation

The parents of young children suffer in this respect. Forty per cent of them consider their children under the age of 4 to have a significant sleeping problem. These parents are 'on call' twenty-four hours a day, week after week, year after year. They will be interested (or dismayed!) to know that the brain cells which initiate their waking sequence are specifically tuned to the noise created by their children. The sound frequencies which they emit are given priority status by the brain. This ensures that the slightest whimper from a child will still manage to wake its mother, whereas a passing train may shake the house but will not disturb her — especially if she is catching up on lost sleep. There is no doubt in my mind that some of these wakeful children are so because of food intolerance.

Case histories

Betty, for example, was at her wits' end. She was the exhausted 32-year-old mother of two. She came to see me when I was still in general practice, and when my interest in allergy was just developing. She asked me for a tonic to give her a 'lift'. She felt irritable with the kids and depressed in herself. On her lap sat a fairly angelic-looking one-year-old child! After discussing the situation, it became clear that a tonic for Betty would have been pointless — it was the child who needed treatment: 'Oh, he's fine,' she said, 'he just doesn't sleep much!' She had had to get up for him a few times every night since he was born. Neither was he happy during the day. She described him as 'always cranky and wanting to be held'. On a purely try-it-and-see basis, the little lad was taken off all dairy produce. A fortnight later, when the case was reviewed, Betty was able to report that she had a 'completely different child'. He smiled by day and slept by night. As for herself, she was sleeping properly for the first time in a year, and felt the benefit of it. She did not need a tonic now because her energy was returning to normal. She was calmer and lighter in mood. I wish that every sleepless child would respond to dietary manipulations of this sort, but they don't. Two of our own children had sleeping problems, or should I say, we considered them to have sleeping problems — they seemed quite happy about it!

One of the worst cases of parental sleep deprivation I have come across is Dorothy. She came to see me at the age of 41 with a complaint of sheer exhaustion. Her problems started sixteen years previously with the birth of her first child. The baby was very active and hardly ever slept: on a good night, Dorothy would get three hours' sleep. Within two months she was depressed, apprehensive and nauseated. The public health nurse called in one day to check on whether Dorothy had any problems with the baby. 'The baby's fine. It's me who has the problem', she said. The baby was examined and found to be normal. Unfortunately, and in spite of the fact that postnatal depression should have been suspected, her plea for help was ignored, and the situation was allowed to deteriorate over the next three years. By then, she felt exhausted and utterly dejected. She suffered daily panic attacks and had lost all confidence in herself. She had also developed a multitude of other symptoms: widespread aches and pains, profuse sweats, diarrhoea and mouth ulcers. Although her child slept from the age 4, Dorothy was never able to restore her own sleep pattern, so she was prescribed antidepressants and tranquillisers. These did not help her at all. Her first-born is now 16 years old, a normal healthy girl in every respect. Dorothy, on the other hand, is far from healthy. She has suffered the devastating consequences of chronic sleep deprivation.

Occupational sleep deprivation

Occupational sleep deprivation is the result of excessive or unusual hours. Shift workers, for instance, are more likely to complain of fatigue and sleepiness than their fellow workers. They have to change 'time zones' frequently, and in the process suffer what may be considered a form of 'occupational jet lag', i.e. a disorganised circadian rhythm. Some 30 per cent of the workforce are simply unable to adjust to these frequent lags and may be described as constitutionally unsuited to shift work — a fact ignored by most employers. The others cope better, but the bottom line is that nobody ever fully adjusts to working all night and sleeping all day. Bats may be nocturnal animals, but humans are not.

Now spare a thought for our junior hospital doctors. They have to work exceptionally long hours, sometimes being on call for 120 hours a week! It is not unusual for them to put in a full weekend of very intensive work on a few hours of broken sleep. Now that you are aware of the implications of this to coherent thought and reliable decision-making, how will you feel the next time you are rushed to hospital for emergency treatment in the early hours of a Monday morning? Sleep deprivation becomes a very serious thing when, as happened, a surgeon falls asleep on his patient in the middle of a major operation; or when yet another driver leaves the road at 70 m.p.h., sleeping peacefully on the steering wheel, never to wake up again. In fact, even professional drivers consistently underestimate the amount of sleep they need. Twenty-five per cent of them are under the dangerous illusion that they only need six hours' sleep per night, or less, relying on caffeine to keep them alert — it doesn't work!

Travellers across time zones are also familiar with this feeling of jet lag. They are well advised not to make important decisions until they have become accustomed to their new schedule. It will take at least twenty-four hours for the circadian rhythm to be restored and brain function to return to normal.

In summary, then, it is clear that we cannot afford to underestimate the consequences to health of sleep deprivation, whatever the cause. To state the obvious, and without wishing to patronise, your first responsibility, if you complain of fatigue, is to revise your sleeping habit. You cannot burn the proverbial candle at both ends and hope to get away with it. Even the most intelligent people underestimate their sleep requirements. Thankfully, it is possible to catch up on lost sleep. In doing so, the brain will spend more time in SW sleep until the deficit has been fully restored. If you are one who needs more sleep, make sure you get it. It may be worth your while to adopt a different use of the alarm clock for a while: depend on it to get you *into* bed, not out of it!

11 *Sleep Disorders*

Insomnia

So much for keeping regular hours; but what if you are unable to sleep? What if you are suffering from insomnia? This is defined as a difficulty initiating or maintaining sleep, in other words, trouble getting to sleep and/or staying asleep. Insomnia is by far the most common sleep disorder. Strictly speaking, we should think of insomnia as either primary (existing in isolation and in its own right) or secondary (the result of some other condition). Fifteen to 25 per cent of all patients with chronic insomnia are diagnosed as having the primary variety. The remaining 75 to 85 per cent have secondary insomnia.

Primary insomnia

We all suffer from insomnia from time to time. There is nothing unusual about this. Knowing we have to get up early to catch a flight, sleeping with 'one ear open' listening for a sick child, or worrying about the next day at work are fairly common experiences. These are examples of anxious thought intruding on slow wave sleep. If the insomnia persists for one month, and if it is not secondary to some other disorder, we refer to it as primary insomnia. Patients may have the impression that they were 'tossing and turning' throughout the night. They may feel that their sleep is useless, that it is 'too light', and that it does nothing to refresh them. These individuals are now at risk of becoming anxious about their sleep. They become physiologically and psychologically aroused worrying about it, and this only serves to worsen their chances of sleep. The harder they try to sleep, the

89

more depressed and frustrated they become — trying to sleep is counterproductive. If the insomnia persists, it leads to fatigue, low mood, loss of energy and motivation, poor concentration and feelings of general malaise. Some individuals will also suffer from tension headache, muscle pain and digestive problems. Transient insomnia may be safely treated with sleeping tablets, but established primary insomnia is probably best treated by cognitive behavioural therapy (page 274-5).

Secondary insomnia

Secondary insomnia is not considered an illness in itself, but rather an indication of other problems, whether physical, psychological or social. In one study, 85 per cent of patients with insomnia were found to be suffering from anxiety and/or depression (these topics are discussed in Section 2). Physical conditions may also interfere with sleep. Pain, for example, is bound to prevent good sleep. Similarly, heartburn, shortness of breath or any number of other symptoms will need to be treated to ensure that they do not disrupt sleep. However, remember that medicines can also interfere. The chief culprits here are the decongestants and steroids, but sometimes the medicines used to treat asthma, high blood pressure and (paradoxically) depression can have the same insomniac effect.

Thus, the treatment of secondary insomnia should always be directed at the underlying cause. The use of sleeping tablets in this context is less helpful. They may actually worsen your fatigue and induce depression (particularly if you are feeling low to start with). They are also addictive, which means that in time you will need more to do the same job. You could run into trouble trying to get off them.

It is worth repeating here that one cause of secondary insomnia is virtually always forgotten, namely, food intolerance. Betty's little boy was a case in point. His insomnia was fully and immediately corrected by the exclusion of all dairy produce from his diet. Adults with sleeping difficulties may also benefit from this approach, especially if they have other symptoms of food intolerance as well.

Case history

Brendan is a 51-year-old farmer who came to see me because of his long history of headache. He described a sensation of 'awful pressure' building up inside his head, together with a piercing pain through the eyes. At first the attacks came every few months and were relieved by taking aspirin; but over the past four years they had become more frequent and more severe. He now had constant pain, day in and day out. Nothing could shift it. He also had a history of asthma and suffered from irritable bowel symptoms (a condition often associated with food intolerance). He also said that for the past eight years he was sleeping only four hours a night. He went to bed every night at 11.30 p.m. and woke at 3 or 3.30 a.m. and could never get back to sleep. As no medication had eased his headache, and because he had this early morning wakening (which is associated with depression), he was told that he was 'stressed' and was prescribed a cocktail of antidepressants and tranquillisers. These did not help, so he stopped taking them. Within fourteen days of a low allergy diet he was able to report a 90 per cent improvement in his overall condition. His headache was barely there, and he was sleeping through the night till 9 a.m.

Restless legs

Restless legs syndrome is an irritating sleep disorder. It refers to varying degrees of discomfort felt in the legs that can only be relieved by movement. The legs feel tense, on edge, jumpy. The discomfort comes on only when the body is trying to relax, especially in the late evening and at bedtime. The sleeper is just about to doze off, but is constantly prevented from doing so by an urge to move the legs. Sheer exhaustion will eventually drag the victim to sleep, but they may be woken again throughout the night by the same discomfort. Needless to say, this syndrome results in all the symptoms of chronic sleep deprivation. Some patients spend the night walking around the house, unable to settle for even a few minutes.

Case history

Bob suffered terribly in this way. Every evening whilst sitting watching television his legs would start to feel restless. He would have to get up and walk around the room for a while. He would then sit again, but only to be overcome with the same irresistible urge to move after fifteen or twenty minutes. This pattern would continue through the evening until bedtime. Then the restlessness would get even worse. Lying down for as little as two minutes is impossible, so he paces the floor until 3 or 4 a.m. At some point thereafter, he literally falls asleep on his feet, and wakes up on the floor with no recollection of lying down to sleep.

Sometimes, simple lifestyle changes will rectify the problem. Avoidance of exercise, nicotine, caffeine and alcohol in the hours preceding bedtime will often help. If this fails, try the following stretching exercise just before settling down.

Stretching exercise for restless legs

- Stand directly in front of a bedroom wall.
- Raise your arms out straight in front of you, at shoulder height, and put the palms of your hands flat on the wall.
- Shuffle back until the arms are fully outstretched, with the palms still flat on the wall.
- Stand at ease with your arms by your side.
- Take one step further back from the wall.
- Position your feet at shoulder width apart, and keep your heels in contact with the floor throughout.
- Now lean forwards into the wall, with your arms straight out in front of you, until your hands fall flat against the wall.
- Keeping your heels on the ground, bend the arms and lean into the wall as far as you can.
- You should feel a pull in the calf muscles and behind the knees.
- Hold this position for 30 seconds, then relax and walk a short circle.
- Repeat the exercise two or three times before getting into bed.

(This will significantly help 50 per cent of cases.)

Periodic limb movement disorder (PLMD)

Periodic limb movement disorder refers to limb movements that occur during sleep. These may take the form of small muscle twitches or jerks, but they may also be quite sudden and violent. Very often the sleeper is totally unaware of the movement, but their sleeping partner may complain! The latter are sometimes punched and kicked through the night, and carry the bruises throughout the day to prove it. PLMD may occur in isolation or in conjunction with restless legs. Young people may be affected, but it is more common in the elderly. However, it is not necessarily a problem *per se*. A third of people over the age of 65 have the disorder, but only a fraction of these complain of excessive daytime sleepiness or fatigue. PLMD in association with restless legs is much more likely to result in symptoms. In these cases it should be treated, and several drugs are available for this purpose.

Sleep apnoea syndrome

So far we have looked at the problems of getting to sleep, and staying asleep. But sleep is much more than simply falling unconscious and remaining oblivious for the duration of the night. What happens to our sleep architecture during sleep is just as important. Patients with sleep disorders may not be aware of the severe disruption that occurs while they sleep. Remember, we need quality as well as quantity.

Sleep apnoea literally means 'not breathing in sleep'. Obviously, this refers to repeated brief episodes of not breathing during sleep, rather than a total and prolonged cessation of breathing — which would result in death. There are two reasons for a failure to breathe properly: one is mechanical and the other is neurological. Mechanical apnoea is by far the most common, and results from the obstruction of the upper airways by the tissues that surround them. The soft palate, for example, may become elongated and swollen by repeated snoring. Similarly, the tonsils may be too large, or the lower jaw and tongue may be set too far back. Obese individuals are at particular risk because of fatty tissue accumulating in the neck. The net result is that the airway tissues are too floppy.

As air is sucked in with each breath, the soft tissues vibrate off each other, a sound we recognise as a snore. As the muscles relax during sleep, the soft tissues collapse completely and cut off the airway. Carbon dioxide levels then build up, and oxygen levels fall. These are potentially serious biochemical events, and they trigger an alarm in the brain. The brain responds by waking up, for a split second (a micro-arousal), to take what we might call a 'conscious breath'. There may be hundreds of these brief interruptions throughout the night, and they disrupt the sleep pattern profoundly.

However, these micro-arousals are too brief to be remembered in the morning. Thus, the patients themselves are usually unaware of the problem. What they are conscious of is a vague sense of poor quality sleep and excessive daytime sleepiness. They are prone to micro-sleeps throughout the day, i.e. they fall asleep on their feet, for a split second at a time, many times a day. They also complain of poor concentration, irritability, poor memory and low mood. They may experience dull morning headaches and trouble with impotence. Severe cases may even develop high blood pressure, heart disease and stroke. The condition affects 2 to 4 per cent of middle-aged adults, most commonly overweight men.

Classically, it is the spouse who brings attention to the possibility of sleep apnoea. They tell us that the patient snores heavily, and they describe a rather typical sequence of events.

1. They hear the usual thunderous snoring (the floppy airways vibrating together).
2. This suddenly stops (the airways become completely obstructed).
3. Then there is what seems like an age of silence, usually about ten seconds (the apnoea).
4. This is followed by a violent gasp for air (the brain waking up for a conscious breath).
5. The cycle is repeated throughout the night (severely disrupting sleep architecture).

Case history

Sleep apnoea can be both embarrassing and frightening. Take Louise, for example, a 50-year-old mother and teacher. She complained of fatigue for as long as she could remember. In fact, she said that fatigue had 'dogged her entire life'. She claimed that she could fall asleep anywhere, at the drop of a hat, and that she fell asleep before her head touched the pillow at night. These are sure signs of excessive daytime sleepiness. Her husband refused to share a bedroom with her, complaining that she sounded like a sawmill. She ran into similar difficulties when she went on holiday with her friends. However, there was one longstanding girlfriend, Thelma, who described herself as a 'deep sleeper', and wasn't bothered by noise. She stuck with Louise and agreed to share a room — that was until Louise had a prolonged apnoea attack lasting thirty seconds or so. She turned so blue that Thelma thought she was dead; and when she ran over to give her a shake, Louise let out an almighty snort — even more frightening than the apnoea! She refused to share thereafter. Happily, Louise has now been treated and her problem is a thing of the past.

The neurological cause of apnoea is rare. In this case the airways themselves are not obstructed, so snoring is not a feature of this disorder. It is the muscles of respiration, and the central nervous system that drives them, that are at fault. This is called central apnoea. In health, we have an 'automatic breathing control centre' in our brain that keeps us breathing during sleep — we don't have to think about it. If this centre is disrupted by disease, it fails to function properly. The sleeper suffers from the same apnoea attacks and the same micro-arousals through the night. They are often more conscious of disturbed sleep than patients with obstructive apnoea. And although they do not run the same risk of heart disease or stroke, they do suffer from the other symptoms of sleep deprivation. It is, of course, possible to have a mixed apnoea with features of both obstructive and central disorders.

All patients with sleep apnoea are encouraged to avoid alcohol and other sedatives, and to avoid deliberate sleep deprivation, as these will aggravate the condition. Treatment possibilities include the well-known anecdote of changing the sleeping position from flat on the back to lying on one side, but this will help only some patients. Weight loss for the obese is encouraged, but at least 20 kilograms need to be shed before the sleep quality will improve. If these measures fail, then significant improvements can be secured with dental appliances, surgery or artificially assisted respiration.

The latter involves wearing an oxygen mask or nasal prongs during sleep. A special machine delivers air under constant pressure throughout the night. This prevents the floppy tissues from collapsing and keeps the airway open. Special oral appliances may also be tried in an effort to achieve the same goal. The last resort is to submit to surgery of the upper airways. There are several options to consider. The removal of very large tonsils and adenoids may help some, whereas operations to reduce the size of the soft palate may help others. Finally, the more drastic step of creating a hole in the windpipe to bypass the obstruction (a tracheostomy) is reserved for patients with very severe disease who fail to respond to other measures.

Narcolepsy

Case history

Julia is a 24-year-old hairstylist. She gave a very interesting, if distressing, clinical history. She told me that she was perfectly well until she suffered a bad bout of flu some eight years previously, and that she has been constantly unwell since then. She complained of chronic fatigue. However, on closer questioning, her real problem turned out to be one of excessive daytime sleepiness. She said things like, 'I can't get into a car without falling asleep', and 'I could fall asleep standing in a queue.' She admitted falling asleep behind the wheel of her car — and not just once. She tried to fight her sleepiness, but she felt actual pain in trying to do so. Her night time sleep was deep and prolonged, often sleeping from 9 p.m. through till 8 a.m. the next day. She also volunteered that she suffered from bouts of paralysis both at night and during the day. She described sitting in her salon and being suddenly frozen, unable to move, for several minutes at a time. These bouts seemed to be brought on by stress. On occasion, she woke from night time sleep convinced that she had a stroke, with her arms and legs totally paralysed. She would lie there petrified for a few minutes and then, to her great relief, she would be able to move again. She also had hallucinations, frightening visions of things in the room that weren't really there. She thought she was going mad, but she is not. Julia suffers from narcolepsy, in her case possibly brought on by an infection.

Narcolepsy is characterised by irresistible attacks of sudden sleep that are experienced as refreshing, and which occur daily over at least three months. Several attacks (2–6) may occur daily, each one staving off sleepiness for a few hours. In addition, episodes of cataplexy may occur. Cataplexy is experienced as a sudden loss of muscle tone lasting from seconds to minutes and often precipitated by strong emotion such as laughter or anger. Hallucinations, which may occur going into or coming out of sleep, are the result of sudden intrusions of REM (dreaming) sleep into the interval between sleep and wakefulness. Sleep paralysis may occur through the same mechanism.

Narcolepsy affects one in every 2,000 people, but most of these remain undiagnosed for years. This is a pity, because apart from the fact that patients are needlessly embarrassed and baffled by their symptoms, their quality of life can be drastically improved by appropriate medical treatment.

Primary hypersomnia

Case history

Robert was a 21-year-old student, used to a very active social and sporting life and proud of his place on the university football team. At least he was until one year ago, when he got glandular fever. Since then he has been ill. He spent the first five weeks in bed recovering from the effects of a sore throat and swollen glands. The striking feature of his history was this: he was unable to stay awake for any length of time. When I first saw him he was still sleeping around the clock. He would wake, feeling like death warmed up, at 11 a.m. He would then muster all his energy and eventually manage to drag himself out of bed. His legs and arms were sore. He would then sit for an hour or two, listless and sleepy. This was followed by a return to bed and another two or three hours of deep sleep. He still felt dreadful when he woke up. Nevertheless, he would always try to leave the house to visit his girlfriend or his team-mates. He might last an hour or two with these, only to be overcome yet again with a desire for sleep. He had no other symptoms. Robert has hypersomnolence, in his case brought on by a viral infection. We can think of it like this: insomnia is difficulty initiating or maintaining sleep; hypersomnia is difficulty attaining and maintaining wakefulness. They are opposite ends of the spectrum. Robert responded very well to a specific medicine for the disorder.

Hypersomnia is defined as excessive sleepiness over at least one month, severe enough to cause significant distress or functional impairment. Prolonged night time sleep episodes of up to twelve hours' duration may occur, often followed by difficulty waking up. There may also be intentional or inadvertent daytime sleep episodes lasting an hour or more. In contrast to narcolepsy, these are experienced as unrefreshing. Involuntary sleep episodes tend to occur during monotonous, low-stimulation situations, such as watching TV or reading.

Sleep problems in other disorders

It is worth repeating at this stage that sleep disturbance may accompany a large variety of physical and mental illnesses. Specifically, and in the context of chronic fatigue, I would like to draw your attention to a peculiar fact about viruses. We've just seen how viral infections may lead to sleep disorders, but they may also cause depressive illnesses and chronic fatigue states. This means that we cannot jump to conclusions in relation to chronic fatigue syndrome (which often starts with an infection). We cannot say, 'It must be CFS because it started when I got the flu.' It could be, of course, but we should also consider the possibility of a depressive illness or a sleep disorder. Nor is this the only source of error. We know that depressed patients often complain of fatigue, and that fatigued patients often become depressed; and, as if that wasn't enough, that both groups may suffer from sleep disturbance. There is, therefore, considerable scope for confusion here. For the sake of clarity, take a brief look at the sleep disturbance of some of these conditions.

SLEEP PROBLEMS IN DEPRESSION

There are several patterns of sleep disturbance in depression, most commonly insomnia. This may take the form of initial insomnia, where the patient is unable to get off to sleep, but the classical disturbance is of middle or terminal insomnia, that is, patients can usually get off to sleep, but they waken in the middle of the night and have difficulty getting back to sleep; or they waken very early in the morning (e.g. 3 or 4 a.m.) and cannot sleep at all thereafter. This is called early morning wakening. Sometimes the sleep disturbance of depression is the hypersomnolent variety, particularly in atypical depression.

SLEEP PROBLEMS IN ANXIETY

Significant anxiety is virtually always accompanied by insomnia.

SLEEP PROBLEMS IN CHRONIC FATIGUE SYNDROME

Patients with chronic fatigue syndrome frequently have disturbed sleep patterns; so much so that some experts believe that the syndrome is a primary sleep disorder. Many CFS patients are hypersomnolent, some are insomniac, and a few have what is called a circadian disorder. In its worst form, the latter is characterised by not being able to sleep until dawn, and then sleeping solidly until the mid to late afternoon. Correction of the sleep pattern is of the utmost importance in the successful management of CFS. (We will address this issue in detail in Chapter 25.)

SLEEP PROBLEMS IN FIBROMYALGIA

Fibromyalgia is invariably associated with various degrees of insomnia, and insomnia is often the first symptom to appear on the scene. The muscular pain and fatigue that is characteristic of the disorder arises as a direct consequence of the sleep disruption. Obviously, not all insomniacs develop fibromyalgia, so there are undoubtedly other factors involved. We will come back to this in Chapter 21.

A word about sleeping sickness

The term 'sleeping sickness' is sometimes used jokingly to describe a state of fatigue. For your information, sleeping sickness is a tropical parasitic disease transmitted by the tsetse fly. In the final stages of the illness, victims sleep practically all the time.

They even fall asleep during meals and, unless they are constantly woken and fed, they will starve to death.

How do you diagnose a sleep disorder?

If you feel that you may be suffering from a sleep disorder, and if you are failing to progress with simple measures, then your doctor may wish to refer you to a sleep disorders specialist. These doctors run sleep 'laboratories' where your sleep architecture can be studied objectively and in great detail (the polysomnograph).

Getting a good night's sleep

Here are a few simple measures that will improve your sleep quality:

1. Keep a regular schedule.
   - Eat regular meals.
   - Take regular exercise.
   - Get out of bed at the same time every day.
   - Avoid daytime naps, especially if you have trouble sleeping at night.

2. Avoid stimulation in the evening.
   - Don't go to bed hungry or too full.
   - Avoid television and computer screens for one hour before bedtime.
   - Avoid problem-solving late at night.
   - Avoid smoking, caffeine and alcohol.

3. Secure a conducive sleep environment.
   - Quiet (consider ear plugs).
   - Dark (consider shades).
   - Not too hot
   - Not too cold.

4. If you cannot sleep after thirty minutes, get up, move to another room and read in dim light, or listen to soothing music until you are sleepy.
5. Explore the underlying stress and depression of insomnia.

12   *Diet, Mood and Energy*

It is well known that a nutritious diet is essential for optimal physical and mental health. Such a diet would contain adequate amounts of carbohydrate, protein and fat, as well as essential vitamins and minerals. Carbohydrates, proteins and fats are known as macro-nutrients which are packed with energy. The unit of energy we use in relation to food is the kilocalorie, a notion familiar to many. One kilocalorie, by definition, is the amount of energy required to heat one kilogram of water by one degree centigrade. In practice we drop the 'kilo' bit and refer simply to calories. The energy of any food can be measured, for we know:

- One gram of carbohydrate provides 3.75 calories of energy.
- One gram of protein provides 4 calories.
- One gram of fat provides 9 calories.

You can see immediately that fats contain more energy than carbohydrates or protein — and that's why they are, literally, more fattening (hence the expression 'fats make you fat'). Alcohol is also quite fattening as it provides 7 calories per gram. We need to understand that the energy we derive from food is no different from the energy derived from other types of fuel. For example, wheat has been used to power locomotives in times of excessive production, and experiments have shown that the human body can extract almost as much energy from wheat as an engine would. We need this energy for our bodily functions, including muscular movement, breathing, heartbeat, gut motility, nerve function, and so on.

Vitamins and minerals are known as micro-nutrients. These are essential for our well-being, not because they provide energy *per se*, but because they help the body to utilise the energy we get from macro-nutrients. They are also essential for the many biochemical processes that go on in our bodies all the time. Micro-nutrients cannot be manufactured in the human body, so it is essential that they are present in the diet.

The principles of a healthy diet

A healthy diet is all about balance. Too much or too little of anything could lead to nutritional problems. We will discuss the former under the heading of overweight and obesity, and the latter under the heading of nutritional deficiency. But first we will discuss the healthy diet. There is now broad agreement on what constitutes the perfect diet. The principles can be summarised under three convenient headings:

1. Major on the carbohydrates.
2. Go easy on the fats.
3. Eat plenty of fruit and vegetables.

Principle 1: Major on the carbohydrates

Carbohydrate foods should be the main constituent of a properly balanced diet. They should account for 70 per cent of total calories ingested. The main sources of dietary carbohydrate include (i) cereals, (ii) fruit and vegetables, (iii) milk and cheese, and (iv) purified carbohydrates added to foods during manufacture. Dietary carbohydrates are usually considered under two main headings: sugars and polysaccharides. From a human point of view, the most important sugars are:

(a) the single sugar units (monosaccharides), which are
  * glucose
  * galactose
  * fructose
(b) the double sugar units (disaccharides), which are
  * sucrose (glucose and fructose)
  * lactose (glucose and galactose)
  * maltose (glucose and glucose).

Polysaccharides are also further subdivided into

- starches (multiple units of glucose linked together in a chain) and
- non-starch polysaccharides — frequently referred to as 'dietary fibre'.

Glucose is by far the most important of all these sugars. The disaccharides and polysaccharides are broken up in the gut to release their single sugar units. Single units of glucose can be absorbed straight away; all other types of sugar are converted to glucose and then absorbed. The digestion, absorption and transport of carbohydrates are highly regulated processes that combine to achieve and maintain a relatively constant blood glucose level. This ensures a steady supply of glucose to cells around the body. Insulin promotes the entry of glucose into cells, where it is finally metabolised to release energy.

Surplus glucose (not immediately required for energy) is polymerised (linked together) and stored as glycogen in virtually all cells. However, this capacity is limited. Liver and muscle cells may devote 8 and one per cent of their respective total weights to glycogen storage. This glycogen may be quickly broken down to provide glucose if the demand should arise. But once the glycogen storage capacity is reached, the remaining surplus glucose is converted to triglyceride and stored in adipose tissue as fat.

Principle 2: Go easy on the fats

Dietary fats are an essential component of the diet: they are the most energy-dense food available; they carry fat-soluble vitamins; they are involved in cell membrane structure and function; and they are the basic building blocks of many important chemicals and hormones. However, because fats are so energy dense (and taste so nice!) they are an important factor in the development of overweight and obesity. Furthermore, epidemiological studies show that fat consumption is related to death from stroke and heart disease. This effect is directly related to cholesterol levels: for every 0.026 mmol/l increase in cholesterol, there is a 1–2 per cent increased risk of heart disease.

However, not all fats are the same, nor do they all have the same effect on cholesterol. Saturated fats are the most likely to cause problems, because they have a clear cholesterol-raising effect. On the other hand, polyunsaturated fats (also called omega-3 and omega-6 essential fatty acids) do not raise cholesterol levels. This is the reason behind the preference for using polyunsaturated as opposed to saturated fats. A simple rule of thumb is that saturated fats are solid at room temperature (e.g. butter), whereas unsaturated fats are liquid (e.g. olive oil).

For these reasons it is recommended that:

- Fat consumption should be *reduced* to provide no more than 30 per cent of total calorie intake.
- No more than 10 per cent of calories should come from saturated fats.
- The consumption of omega-3 fats (fish) should increase from the present average consumption to 0.2 g per day (equivalent to one tin of sardines every five days).
- The consumption of omega-6 fats should continue at the present rate of consumption.

Principle 3: Eat plenty of fruit and vegetables

A great deal of attention has been paid in recent years to the possible protective effect of certain foods, and particularly those that contain antioxidants. There is reason to believe that fruit and vegetables, which are high in antioxidants, can significantly reduce our risk of heart disease, stroke, cataracts and cancer. For example, there is consistent evidence of an association between high levels of heart disease and low levels of antioxidants, such as vitamin E, vitamin C and the flavanoids. This suggests that people with high intakes of fruit and vegetables (and hence high levels of antioxidants) are protected from heart disease. Similarly, there have been in excess of two hundred studies that strongly suggest an association between a *high* vegetable and fruit intake and a two to four-fold *reduction* in the risk of many cancers. Apart from their protective effects, there are other benefits to increasing our consumption of fruit and vegetables: they are a convenient way of reducing our consumption of fats and a good way to obtain more fibre. All this boils down to one simple piece of advice: we should all be eating at least five portions (400 g) of fruit and vegetables per day.

A word about protein

Although much has been written about protein in relation to physical strength and stamina, the fact is that we need very little protein. Four hundred milligrams per day will meet most people's needs.

The food pyramid

All these principles of a healthy diet have been conveniently simplified in the concept of the food pyramid. If you follow the general guidelines of the pyramid, you will be eating a balanced, nutritious and healthy diet. The basic idea is that foods on the bottom tier of the pyramid can be (and should be) eaten often, whereas foods in the top tier should be eaten sparingly (see diagram).

The food pyramid

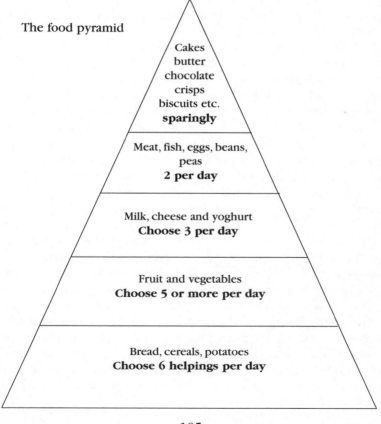

Cakes
butter
chocolate
crisps
biscuits etc.
sparingly

Meat, fish, eggs, beans, peas
2 per day

Milk, cheese and yoghurt
Choose 3 per day

Fruit and vegetables
Choose 5 or more per day

Bread, cereals, potatoes
Choose 6 helpings per day

Diet, mood and well-being

Several dietary factors exert a direct effect on mood and well-being. For example, it has been shown time and again that deficiencies of several nutrients can adversely affect brain function. Vitamin B1 (thiamine), vitamin B6 (pyridoxine), vitamin B12, folate, vitamin C, vitamin D3, selenium and iron all exert independent effects on mood. The usual effect of deficiency is to feel tired and depressed. Indeed, sometimes supplementation with these nutrients produces an improved mood, even in the absence of overt deficiency. For example, some women with premenstrual syndrome report significant therapeutic benefits from vitamin B6. Similarly, improved mood has been attributed to thiamine and selenium supplementation. Other studies have shown that (even clinical) depression is associated with essential fatty acid (omega-3) depletion, and that essential fatty acid supplements can improve the mood of depressed patients. However, too much fat in the diet can lead to sleepiness and fatigue.

It may surprise you to learn that the carbohydrate and protein content of our diet can also affect our mood and energy levels. For example, diets that are high in protein are associated with feelings of depression, tension and anger! Conversely, diets low in carbohydrate are associated with fatigue and depression, whereas high-carbohydrate diets are associated with improved energy and mood. I'll say that again: a higher intake of carbohydrates results in better energy levels and better mood! Carbohydrates are thought to exert their effects by altering neurotransmitter levels in the brain. This is how it works. The central neurotransmitter, serotonin, is made from tryptophan (an amino acid we get from food). Diets high in carbohydrate favour the conversion of tryptophan to serotonin. Conversely, if tryptophan is missing from the diet, serotonin levels fall. Fortunately, profound tryptophan depletion can only be achieved experimentally, so we are not going to suddenly become tryptophan depleted (and suicidal). But what is fascinating, to say the least, is that some of us are particularly prone to the depressive effects of tryptophan depletion, and the rest of us are not. You've guessed it: patients with a history of depression are vulnerable, but so too are their first-degree relatives! This reflects both the biochemical and genetic aspects of depression. This reinforces the assertion that depression is not just 'all in the mind'. As an interesting aside, cosmetic diets (which are low in calories) also lead to a relative tryptophan depletion — have you ever become depressed on a diet?

The enhanced energy and mood effects of a high-carbohydrate diet require a *long-term* strategy. Single meals of carbohydrate do *not* lift the mood; nor do high carbohydrate diets eaten for less than seven days. We are fortunate, then, that long-term high-carbohydrate diets are not only good for us, but they improve our general sense of well-being to boot.

This raises two interesting topics, namely, food craving and comfort eating. Carbohydrate craving has been observed in patients with seasonal affective disorder (SAD, winter depression), *bulimia nervosa*, premenstrual syndrome and the syndrome of carbohydrate-craving obesity. This led some researchers to the hypothesis that these patients were trying (subconsciously) to increase serotonin levels in their brain.

Food craving is closely linked to the phenomenon of comfort eating, and the same theory of serotonin enhancement has been suggested as the underlying mechanism. But research has shown that the 'comfort' we get from eating, say, a bar of chocolate, has more to do with the pleasure of taste and texture than with serotonin levels! We must also remember that cravings may arise in the context of sleep disorders, depression and (occasionally) in food intolerance.

13 *Overweight and Obesity*

It may seem strange to include the subject of overweight and obesity in a book dealing with fatigue, but there are good reasons for doing so. In the first place, overweight individuals who manage to lose weight will report that improved energy levels are one of the first benefits they experience. Gross obesity (defined below) may have a profound adverse effect on energy levels. For this reason, gross obesity is considered an exclusionary disorder in the evaluation of chronic fatigue syndrome. In other words, we cannot diagnose chronic fatigue syndrome in patients who are very obese, because we know that if they lose weight their energy levels will improve.

The second reason for dealing with obesity is that much confusion exists about the role of food allergy and intolerance leading to weight gain, and I would like to address some of these issues.

Let us start by examining our energy requirements. To maintain an ideal body weight we must balance our energy intake with our energy output. When all is said and done, our energy output (and hence our energy requirement) boils down to two simple parameters. These are (1) our basal metabolic rate, and (2) our levels of physical activity.

The basal metabolic rate (BMR) is usually the greatest portion of total energy expenditure over a day, accounting for up to 75 per cent of energy requirement. This is the energy we need to simply stay alive. The biosynthesis of protein, fat and glucose accounts for some 40 per cent of the BMR; active transport across cell membranes accounts for another 38 per cent; and the mechanics of living, such as breathing, heartbeat and intestinal motility etc. make up the remaining 22 per cent. So these are the basic metabolic requirements. But before we can metabolise our food we must first digest and absorb it. These are also energy-dependent processes using up about 10 per cent of the energy of foods eaten. So the next time you reach for a bar of chocolate, you can fool yourself with the thought that 10 per cent of these calories will be used up before you even absorb it — and then try to forget about the other 90 per cent!

How do I estimate my metabolic rate?

Simple equations exist to help you estimate your basal metabolic rate. Your age, gender and weight are used in the formula. You can work out your own BMR by the following table.

Estimating your basal metabolic requirement

	Age	Your BMR in calories equals
Males	10–17 years	(weight in kg x 17.7) + 657
	18–29 years	(weight in kg x 15.1) + 692
	30–59 years	(weight in kg x 11.5) + 873
Females	10–17 years	(weight in kg x 13.4) + 692
	18–29 years	(weight in kg x 14.8) + 487
	30–59 years	(weight in kg x 8.3) + 846

Example: A 43-year-old man who weighs 80 kg would have a BMR of $80 \times 11.5 = 920 + 873 = 1{,}793$ calories per day.

There is some variation in the efficiency with which individuals utilise their food. In practice this means that there may be a difference in energy requirement of plus or minus 10 per cent between one individual and the next. Thus, someone with a very high BMR could require 20 per cent more energy than someone with a very low BMR. So it would be more correct to say that our 43-year-old man has a BMR of 1,793 (+ or – 10%). You will immediately notice that the heavier you are, the higher will be your BMR. So the contention that 'I am fat because I have a slow metabolism' is patently false. The fact is, the heavier you are, the greater is your metabolic rate! As can be clearly seen, we gain weight because we eat more energy than we burn up — and for no other reason.

Physical activity

Physical activity requires energy over and above the BMR. Even the most sedentary have a minimum physical activity level which increases their requirement by 25 to 35 per cent. If they happen to be restless and fidgety, they may burn up a further 800 calories each day. The very active may increase their total energy requirement by a factor of two; and with intense physical training it is possible to increase expenditure to many times the BMR. Thus, it is clear that the level of physical activity is a very important factor in determining an individual's energy requirement. Finally, certain groups, such as growing children, pregnant and lactating mothers, athletes, and the ill or convalescent have special energy requirements.

Why do we gain weight and grow fat?

Our bodies are very efficient in terms of handling the energy we ingest. If we eat more energy than we use up, our bodies will store the excess energy in fat cells. It does not matter if the energy has been consumed as fat, alcohol, carbohydrate or protein, for these are all converted into fat for storage. This storage facility has been extremely useful historically, especially in times of hardship. Thus, when food was abundantly available (typically during summer time), we could eat to our hearts' content and put on a little weight in the process. We would then have had a store of energy to keep us going during the long winter months when food was not so readily available. Thus we would pass through cycles of weight gain followed by weight loss, and we would maintain a healthy body weight year on year. The unpredictability of food supplies is still a major problem in many parts of the world today. But those of us who are blessed with affluence no longer have to face harsh winters. That means we no longer get the chance to shed a few pounds every year. As a result, we store more and more fat in our fat cells.

Incidentally, we all have fat cells, even the thinnest among us, so the difference between those who are thin and those who are overweight is the amount of fat stored in their fat cells. It is quite remarkable that, in spite of all the variables mentioned above, most of us regulate our energy intake quite naturally with an error margin of less than one per cent over a lifetime.

This is true even for the very obese. Gluttony is a rare cause of obesity, yet the obese are regarded with the suspicion that they are just greedy. Not so! They have made a very slight error, that's all. Unfortunately, it is an error which accumulates over the years as flab. This is worth a closer look. Even tiny amounts of energy can add up over the years to significant weight gain. For example, if you consume eight calories per day more than you use up, you will put on twenty pounds weight in as many years. Think of it this way: fat is energy stored. Each pound of fat contains 3,000 calories of energy, so if you are twenty pounds overweight, you have a store equivalent to 60,000 calories. Divide that by 7,300 days (20 years) and you come up with the figure of eight calories per day. Come back now to our 43-year old who had a basal metabolic requirement of 1,793 calories per day. And let's give him a modest level of physical activity, say, 25 per cent. His total energy requirement would now be 2,241 calories (1,793 + 25% of 1,793). If he had eaten only eight calories per day more than he should have, that would be an error rate of 0.36 per cent, or one spoonful of breakfast cereal per day! It's as simple as that, and as you can see, it has nothing whatsoever to do with food allergy or intolerance. These are basic laws of biology.

In order to lose weight then, we simply need to reduce our intake and/or increase our output. This is seldom mentioned in the plethora of diet theories available today. There should be equal emphasis on intake and output, that is, equal attention should be paid to diet and exercise. As mentioned above, exercise greatly increases our energy output. For example, if you were to increase your output every day by walking for an hour, you would burn off 240 calories x 365 days = 87,600 calories per year, which is equivalent to 29 pounds of fat! Go for it!

How do I know if I'm too fat?

There is a very simple way to assess your weight. It's called the body mass index (BMI). This is how you calculate your BMI:

- Weigh yourself in kilograms.
- Measure your height in metres.
- Multiply your height by itself (height squared).
- Divide your weight by your height squared.
- The result is your BMI.

Example:
Let's say your height is 1.74 meters, and your weight is 90 kilograms. Multiply your height by itself: 1.74 x 1.74 = 3.0276. Now divide your weight (90) by 3.0276. Your BMI is 29.7. What does that mean? It means you are overweight. The ideal BMI is anywhere from 20 to 25. This takes account of your age, your sex and your bone structure etc. In other words, there are no excuses! A BMI between 25 and 30 is the current definition of 'overweight', and a BMI greater than 30 is the current definition of 'obesity'.

Does it matter if I'm too fat?

Overweight and obesity are strongly associated with ill health, and that's why doctors go on about the importance of losing weight. For instance, the overweight have a greater incidence of diabetes, high blood pressure, stroke, heart disease, respiratory disease, cancer, gall stones, arthritis, varicose veins, hernias, and even accidents! To put it bluntly, a BMI of 34 is associated with a 50 per cent increase in mortality, and a BMI of 36 is associated with a two-fold increase in mortality. (The heavier you are, the greater your risk of an early death.) These figures have come from large life assurance companies. They are keen to load the premiums of obese people because they know there is a greater chance of having to make an early payment! However, it is not just a question of being heavy. Studies which examined the fitness levels of the obese have found that obesity *per se* is not the risk factor; it's the lack of physical fitness. Thus, a very fit obese person is less likely to die young than a sedentary thin person. This suggests that being overweight merely reflects the relative inactivity of the vast majority of obese individuals. The message to take from all this is a positive one: don't just sit there, do something!

14 Nutritional Deficiency

The most devastating form of nutritional deficiency is, of course, starvation, and this may be partial or complete. Even milder partial forms of starvation will result in growth retardation, developmental delay, increased susceptibility to infection and decreased work performance. More severe and prolonged starvation will give rise to the clinical conditions known as kwashiorkor and marasmus, pictures of which we have all seen on our television screens.

But these and other full-blown nutritional diseases such as beriberi (vitamin B1 deficiency) or scurvy (vitamin C deficiency) are seldom seen in the developed countries, except when they occur as a consequence of some other major disorder such as cancer, alcoholism or anorexia (from whatever cause). We may be thereby deceived into believing that nutritional deficiency is a problem encountered only in the developing countries, but this is far from true. It is important to remember that the absence of a severe nutritional deficiency is *not* proof of adequate nutrition, and that the aim of good nutrition is not just the prevention of a nutritional disaster. Rather, it has much to do with attaining and maintaining *optimal* health.

Less severe nutritional deficiencies can and do arise in our so called 'well-fed' societies, and much more commonly than has previously been supposed. In these less severe deficiency states, patients do not demonstrate all the features of full-blown malnutrition, but they do feel unwell none the less. Fatigue is commonly experienced in this context, and so in this chapter we will take a closer albeit brief look at those deficiencies which most commonly contribute to this complaint.

You may find it hard to believe that there are nutritional deficiencies in an affluent society. To establish that there are, we need only consider the findings of a National Diet and Nutrition Survey, recently carried out in the UK. The authors found cause for concern in many categories, including pre-school children, adults and the elderly.

Malnutrition in pre-school children

Significant numbers of toddlers aged between 1½ and 4½ years have poor vitamin and mineral status:

- 50 per cent have poor vitamin A status.
- 95 per cent have a poor intake of vitamin D.
- 84 per cent have a low intake of iron.
- One in twelve are anaemic.
- 72 per cent have low zinc.
- Up to 68 per cent are low in copper.
- Up to 5 per cent are low in iodine.

Malnutrition in adults

The two major nutritional concerns in adults are:

(1) the increasing incidence of obesity in both sexes.

The prevalence of obesity has increased over the past decade to 16 per cent of women and 13 per cent of men. The percentage of total energy intake derived from fats is unadvisedly high at around 40 per cent, with 16.5 per cent derived from saturated fats.

Note: obesity is a form of malnutrition.

(2) poor iron status in women.

The iron status of fertile women has been found wanting. Studies in this group suggest that

- iron intake is too low.
- blood levels of iron are low in a third of women.
- 4 per cent are anaemic.

Malnutrition in the elderly

There is much concern over micro-nutrient status in the elderly, particularly among those who live in institutions, and worse again in those who are edentate (have no teeth):

- 45 per cent have poor iron status.
- 41 per cent have poor vitamin C status.
- 39 per cent are low in folate.
- 37 per cent are low in vitamins D and B2.
- 9 per cent are low in vitamin B12.
- 13 per cent are low in vitamin B1.

The data for the free-living elderly are somewhat better, but there is still major concern:

- 10 per cent are low in iron.
- 13.5 per cent are low in vitamin C.
- 15 per cent are low in folate.
- 41 per cent are low in vitamin B2.
- 8 per cent are low in vitamin D.
- 6 per cent are low in thiamine.
- 9 per cent are low in vitamin B12.

Why do nutritional deficiencies arise in well-fed societies?

You may well wonder how nutritional deficiencies could possibly occur in well-fed societies. The main reasons are:

- Persistent socio-economic disadvantage in some groups.
- Loss of nutritional value from food as it passes through the food chain.
- Failure to eat a healthy diet in spite of the availability of good food.
- Increased nutritional requirements of certain individuals.

Socio-economic influences on nutritional status

There is evidence to suggest that significant differences exist in food intake patterns between the social classes. In general, social classes IV and V have less dietary variety, with a lower intake of wholegrain foods, vegetables and dietary fibre, and a lower intake of antioxidant foods, when compared to social classes I and II. The poorer classes also have less physical activity and a greater prevalence of obesity. This is supported by the finding that 25 per cent of women and 17 per cent of men in social class V have a BMI greater than 30, compared to 14 and 11 per cent, respectively, in social class I.

The lack of diversity in the low-income diet has adverse effects on nutrient profiles in general. The intake of calcium, iron, magnesium, B vitamins (and folate) and vitamin C are generally lower than in more affluent households. Furthermore, there is special concern for vulnerable groups within low-income families. These include:

- Infants, who are less likely to be breast fed, are more likely to become iron deficient and at greater risk of infection.
- Pre-school children, who have generally poorer diets and slower growth.
- Schoolchildren, especially girls, who have a lower intake of iron and calcium.
- Pregnant women, who have a lower weight gain in pregnancy, lower birth weight babies, more anaemia, and a higher risk of neural tube defects (spina bifida).
- The elderly, who have greater morbidity and mortality from diet-related disease.

Effects on health status

These socio-economic factors contribute significantly to poor nutritional status. The health of members of low-income households is generally poor: they are at greater risk of high blood pressure, heart disease and various cancers. They are also more prone to respiratory and digestive system disorders.

The loss of nutritional value from food

Ideally, a balanced and varied diet should provide us with all our nutritional needs. But it will not do so if the foods we eat have lost some, or most, of their nutritional value. Essential nutrients may be lost from the original food as it passes through the various stages of the food chain. This chain starts in the soil in which the food is grown. From here, the food is harvested, processed and stored. It is eventually distributed to the consumer, who often stores the food again. It has then to withstand the rigours of cooking before finally ending up on the plate.

FOOD PRODUCTION AND PROCESSING

Large-scale food production has led, in some cases, to mineral-depleted soil. Vegetables grown in these soils will be *ipso facto* mineral deficient. Similarly, fruit which is not allowed to ripen on the tree, or which is 'forced' to grow fast, will not produce its full quota of nutrients. For example, oranges picked when they are still green (and most of them are) contain little vitamin C. Further nutritional loss occurs during some food-processing techniques, such as the refining of wheat flour, in which vitamins and minerals are removed along with the unwanted components of the original grain. The addition of man-made chemicals to food may also interfere with its nutrients. Sulphites, for example, used as preservatives, are known to destroy vitamins.

STORAGE, DISTRIBUTION AND COOKING

As soon as a food is harvested from its parent plant, it begins to lose its nutritional value. The longer it takes the food to reach the consumer, the poorer will be its nutritional content. It is therefore important to eat food while it is still fresh. Diets consisting mainly of processed foods are likely to be less nutritious than those containing plenty of fresh food. Even more value is lost during storage and cooking: the longer it is stored, and the harder it is cooked, the less nutritious it will be.

Inadequate dietary intake

As we have seen, the poorer people in our society find themselves unable to afford the healthier foods that are available. However, some people eat wholly inadequate diets, not so much out of financial constraint, but for the sake of convenience or preference. I refer to the all too common practice of surviving mostly on crisps and chocolate bars, or tea and biscuits. (Three million units of a well-known chocolate bar are eaten every day in the UK — and that's only one single product from one manufacturer!)

Some patients, in desperation, put themselves on severely restricted diets in the hope of obtaining relief from various symptoms. Unfortunately, they usually do so without adequate nutritional or medical advice. Those who consider themselves to be allergic to a wide range of foods are prominent in this group. They exclude every food they suspect of causing them trouble and, in so doing, they may be left with only one or two 'safe' foods. I have seen one patient who was eating a diet consisting entirely of potato and polished rice — for breakfast, dinner and tea! Another man had similarly restricted his diet to brown bread and butter. (I will come back to this in Chapter 15.) Finally, those who eat vegetarian, vegan or other restricted diets are also at risk of nutritional deficiency. It goes without saying that *anorexia nervosa* leads to severe and sometimes life-threatening malnutrition.

Increased nutritional requirements

Some physical conditions are complicated by the poor absorption of essential nutrients. Coeliac disease is an example of this. The intestine is damaged by gluten-containing foods and the absorption of nutrients is impaired. This disease is a well-recognised clinical entity and, as such, sufferers are usually given appropriate dietary advice. Other conditions which may have a similar effect are not always recognised as a potential problem, for example, allergic enteritis (inflammation of the intestine) or irritable bowel syndrome. At other times the problem is not one of absorption but of excessive loss. Diabetics, for instance, are frequently low in magnesium, and patients with diarrhoea may lose excessive potassium (see below). But nutritional requirements will increase dramatically in the presence of any disease state, acute or chronic. Take the case of eczema: severely affected children may suffer growth retardation, and adults may suffer from chronic fatigue, unless the condition is properly controlled. Clearly, the recommended daily allowance of essential nutrients, which is based on the average healthy adult or child, is wholly inappropriate for those who have a long-term illness.

Nutritional needs are also greater in athletes, growing children, pregnant or breast feeding women, and during times of emotional stress. Finally, certain medicines (such as the oral contraceptive pill, diuretics and some of the anticonvulsants) interfere with the absorption, utilisation and excretion of nutrients.

Some specific nutritional deficiencies (with specific reference to fatigue)

Vitamin C deficiency

Profound vitamin C deficiency causes scurvy, a condition characterised by fatigue, malaise and weakness, as well as anaemia, gum disease, spontaneous bleeding and easy bruising. It results in a lowered resistance to infection, delayed wound-healing and pains in the bones and joints. Scurvy is now a rare disease in the developed world, but milder forms of deficiency are common. The first symptom is fatigue, and this may be present without any of the other features of scurvy. Furthermore, it is thought that some patients may become depressed or hypochondriacal in thought when they are vitamin C deficient. Deficiency will be prevented by eating such foods as blackcurrants, guavas, rosehip, green peppers, oranges (which have been allowed to ripen on the tree), cauliflower, broccoli, sprouts, cabbage, potato and liver.

Vitamin B deficiency

It is rare to come across an isolated vitamin B deficiency in the developed countries, but there are two exceptions to this. Firstly, alcoholics may develop a serious brain and nerve dysfunction called Wernicke's disease, caused by vitamin B1 (thiamine) deficiency, the consequence of drinking excessive amounts of alcohol, together with a failure to eat nutritious meals. The second exception is that of vitamin B12, which has specific requirements for absorption from the intestine into the blood. If these requirements are not met, deficiency will follow, causing pernicious anaemia — even when adequate amounts of B12 are present in the diet. Because isolated vitamin B deficiencies are rare, and for the sake of simplicity, I will not go into the details of each individual B vitamin. Instead, I will consider the group as a whole. They share many chemical similarities and are found in the same types of food: liver and muscle meats, milk, eggs, whole cereal grains, yeast and green leafy vegetables.

It is obvious then that a diet lacking in one of the B vitamins will almost certainly be lacking in the others also. In any case, the results of deficiency are similar for each B vitamin, so it can be difficult to distinguish, on clinical grounds alone, which one of the B vitamins is responsible for a given symptom. For example, a deficiency of *any* of the B vitamins may cause weakness and fatigue, and these symptoms will develop within a few short weeks of eating a poor diet.

Other symptoms of vitamin B deficiency include:

- dry and peeling lips
- cracks in the corners of the mouth
- a swollen, red or sore tongue
- red greasy skin, especially on either side of the nose and on other parts of the face
- the skin elsewhere may feel rough and itchy.

Nerve cells are particularly sensitive to vitamin B deficiency. If brain cells are deprived, they will give rise to depression, insomnia, irritability, poor memory, confusion and headaches. If the peripheral nerves (which carry messages to and from the brain) are deprived, this will give rise to numbness, pins and needles, burning sensations and paralysis. Serious damage may occur to nerves if adequate supplements are not given in time. A deficiency of folic acid (another B vitamin) or vitamin B12 will result in anaemia, with the usual attendant symptoms, including marked fatigue.

Iron deficiency

Iron deficiency anaemia is covered on pages 60–61. Briefly stated, the symptoms of iron deficiency include marked fatigue, shortness of breath, palpitations, irritability, pins and needles, headache and light-headedness. A sore tongue and cracks at the corners of the mouth may also occur. However, milder forms of iron deficiency are quite common. In these cases you may suffer from fatigue, but without the tell-tale anaemia. Affected subjects experience a reduction in the work capacity of their muscles, resulting in weakness; and children suffer a reduction in their learning ability.

Potassium deficiency

Potassium depletion is an important but lesser known mineral (salt) deficiency. It usually occurs as a result of the excessive loss of potassium from the body. This loss may occur through the bowel (in faeces) or through the kidney (in urine). The most common cause of potassium loss is acute gastroenteritis. In this situation, potassium literally pours out of the bowel, together with vast quantities of sodium and faecal fluid. This accounts in part for the profound weakness that accompanies such an illness. It is imperative that fluid is replaced along with glucose, sodium chloride (table salt) and potassium, in correct proportions.

Fortunately, acute bowel infections like this do not last long. The potassium loss, once it has been corrected, should not therefore recur. But there are a number of chronic bowel diseases that allow varying amounts of potassium to leak from the body over prolonged periods of time (e.g. the inflammatory bowel diseases, ulcerative colitis and Crohn's disease). Not only do these prevent the absorption of essential nutrients, but they also cause potassium loss, which may at times be very severe indeed. The chronic diarrhoea of irritable bowel syndrome, which is more common by far, may cause a similar problem.

Potassium depletion may also occur following the use of certain potassium-losing diuretics (the thiazide and loop diuretics). These medicines have a direct effect on the kidneys, causing them to lose potassium. The patient's blood should be checked at intervals to ensure that adequate levels of potassium are maintained. Finally, potassium depletion may occur as a result of eating too much liqorice! The liqorice present in the bowel will bind to the potassium and prevent its absorption into the bloodstream.

One of the main symptoms of potassium depletion is fatigue. Muscle cramps, depression and loss of appetite also occur; and if the blood levels fall too low, the heart will beat irregularly and may even stop beating altogether. Foods rich in potassium include fresh fruit, vegetables, whole grains and salt substitutes.

Magnesium

Magnesium is essential for healthy muscles and nerves. The consequences of profound magnesium depletion are devastating. When the blood level drops too low, the brain and heart become increasingly irritable. This results in epileptic seizures, tetany (muscle cramps) and irregular heart rhythms which may prove fatal. Because of this, the body will maintain a normal level of magnesium for as long as it possibly can. It does so by drawing magnesium out of other body compartments into the blood. Thus, a low blood level indicates a very severe shortage of the mineral. It signifies that there are little or no magnesium stores left in the body to draw upon. This is a life-threatening state. Blood levels of magnesium are therefore a poor indication of less severe forms of deficiency, in which the cells of the body have donated their magnesium to maintain the blood level, but at their own expense. More accurate assessments of magnesium status are still being sought. One possibility is to measure the levels present inside the circulating red or white blood cells, but even these are subject to error.

Magnesium is widely distributed in many staple foods, such as cocoa, nuts, soya, barley, corn, wheat and oats. Any reasonable diet should therefore contain plenty of it. But deficiency may still occur in a number of situations. Diabetics, patients on diuretics or certain antibiotics or who drink excessive amounts of alcohol will have an increased urinary loss of magnesium. Furthermore, people who use diets which are high in protein, calcium, phosphorus or vitamin D will have an increased dietary requirement of magnesium. Similarly, eating a lot of bran prevents the absorption of magnesium because it becomes bound to the phytates contained therein.

The symptoms of magnesium deficiency are anxiety, irritability, insomnia, depression, muscular pain and fatigue — to name but a few. Some of these symptoms may be due to a functional vitamin B1 or B6 deficiency: magnesium is essential for the efficient utilisation of these vitamins, and when it is not present in sufficient quantity, the vitamins are unable to do their job.

Zinc

Zinc is also widely distributed in many foods, including oysters, meats, nuts, milk, egg, wheat, rye, oats, soy, potato and corn. In spite of this ready availability of zinc, a number of studies have found that adults and children alike are frequently eating less than the recommended daily allowance. Some diuretics, alcohol and high-fibre diets may also produce zinc depletion. Symptoms of deficiency include frequent infections, dry skin, delayed wound-healing, hair loss and fatigue.

Achieving good nutritional status

In the last few chapters we have covered a lot of material. Much of it may be new to you and some of it may be confusing. How do you ensure that you are getting the correct amount of energy, the right kind of fat and plenty of vitamins and minerals? You can achieve all this by following the food pyramid. If you are overweight, increase your exercise rate and reduce your intake a little. Thereafter, simply incorporate the pyramid into your routine. It will soon become second nature to you.

A word of warning

Nutritional deficiency requires specific treatment. Each patient should be assessed individually to determine nutritional status. Many people take it upon themselves to top up with supplements. For the vast majority there is no problem with this, but be careful not to overdose yourself. It is possible to make yourself very sick with vitamin excess. If you are in any doubt, get expert advice.

15 Food Allergy and Intolerance

Allergy and intolerance are vast subjects. In this chapter we will focus particularly on their role in fatigue states. A comprehensive and detailed account of the full range of allergic symptoms is presented in *Could it be an Allergy?*

Case history

Ann Marie is a 35-year-old woman whose problem with fatigue started rather suddenly some two years before I first saw her. She had always enjoyed good health, apart from the postnatal depression which she had after each of her three deliveries. However, with her youngest child now aged 6, and all traces of depression long since passed, she decided to set up her own business as an interior decorator. She coped quite well for the first twelve months with this new venture, but she then hit a brick wall of exhaustion. In addition to 'this dreadful tiredness', she complained of low mood, frequent headaches, fitful sleep and itchy eyes.

It would have been easy to attribute these symptoms to stress or depression: she was rather low in mood, she has a past history of depression, and she has been under considerable stress for a protracted period of time. Ann Marie was well aware of the psychological background to her symptoms, but was also intrigued with her own discovery that certain foods made her feel worse. Wheat leaves her exhausted and sugar-laden foods make her feel drowsy, but potato has the most profound effect of all — within one hour of eating it, she is overcome with an irresistible fatigue from which she cannot recover without first falling asleep!

Hippocrates (460–359 B.C.) was the first physician to describe adverse reactions to food. He said, for example, that although cheese is an excellent food for most, the smallest piece could make some people ill. He had no idea *why* cheese made some people ill, only that it *did*. His approach was, therefore, simple and pragmatic. He made his diagnosis on the grounds of clinical observation alone: if the symptoms under investigation were relieved by avoiding a certain food, and returned again whenever that food was eaten, he would have advised his patient not to eat that food again. The essence of this truth was later captured by the Roman poet Lucretius (94–55 B.C.) with the words: 'One man's meat is another man's poison.'

The term 'allergy' did not come into use until early in the twentieth century when an Austrian physician (von Pirquet) first coined the phrase to describe the serious and sometimes fatal (anaphylactic) reactions which certain children had to vaccination injections. They had developed what he called an 'altered (*allos*) reaction (*ergo*)', or allergy, to the horse serum contained in the vaccines.

Immediate allergic reactions to food

The nature of these immediate reactions was not fully understood until the discovery, in the 1960s, of a specialised protein within the immune system, called immuno-globulin E (IgE). IgE was identified as being responsible for initiating the cascade of allergic events which occur in susceptible individuals, once they have been exposed to their allergens (an allergen being any substance — eaten, inhaled or touched — which provokes an allergic response).

IgE-mediated events are called type 1 allergic reactions. Well-known examples include hay fever (allergy to pollen), urticaria (itchy rash), angioedema (swelling of the soft tissues) and asthma (constriction of the airways). The main feature of type 1 allergies is that they usually produce an *immediate reaction* — so much so that patients have often made their own diagnosis before they see the doctor. 'Every time I eat eggs, I break out in a rash.'

Because of the speed of these reactions, there is seldom any dispute over the diagnosis. Furthermore, they may be confirmed objectively by both skin and blood tests. The skin test is quite simple and may be carried out on the spot in the consulting room. A small drop of the suspected allergen is placed on the forearm, and the underlying skin is pricked with a lancet. If a wheal (a red itchy lump) develops at the site within ten minutes or so, the patient is said to be allergic to that substance. The blood test, on the other hand, is carried out in the laboratory, where a quantitative measurement of IgE is made, and where the allergens against which the IgE is directed are identified. For example, if the blood is found to contain significant amounts of IgE directed against egg, then that patient is, without a shadow of doubt, allergic to egg. Strangely, this patient may not yet have symptoms when exposed to egg, in which case the allergy is described as latent or dormant. But the potential for an allergic reaction is very much present.

It is thought that somewhere between one and two per cent of the population suffers from type 1 food allergy. A small number of these are exquisitely sensitive to their allergens. They can experience dramatic, frightening and sometimes life-threatening reactions after even the slightest allergen exposure. Such is the case with 2-year-old Paul. His face and mouth begin to swell if he so much as *handles* an egg — I dread to think what would happen if he ate one! Similarly, 17-year-old James starts to wheeze if he walks past the fish counter in the supermarket — the *smell* (air-borne molecules of fish allergen) being sufficient to initiate allergic symptoms.

Patients who have life-threatening reactions should always carry an adrenaline syringe on their person for emergency use. Adrenaline is a very effective and life-saving treatment which reverses all the symptoms and thus controls the reaction within minutes of injection — an injection which patients can easily administer to themselves. Deaths *have* occurred as a result of severe allergic reactions to food. It is difficult to obtain precise figures on this, but at least 150 people die in European Union member states each year from anaphylaxis, and possibly as many as 8,500 per annum in the USA. The tragedy is that most of these deaths could have been avoided. In the first place, the patients concerned were not fully aware of the various ways in which they could possibly stumble upon their culprit foods when these were disguised in prepared meals — who would expect to find walnuts in a lamb stew, for instance? Secondly, they were usually caught without their adrenaline syringe, so that when they did accidentally eat an allergen, they were without their most effective treatment. One man who knew that he was allergic to peanuts, started to wheeze during a Chinese meal which was flavoured with Satay sauce. Unfortunately, he did not know that Satay sauce is made from peanuts. He died on his way back to the hotel where he had left his adrenaline syringe. Another patient, equally aware of her allergy to peanuts, died within minutes of eating a vegetarian burger which was laden with this food. It is worth repeating: those who have life-threatening reactions should *always* carry an adrenaline injection on their person for emergency use.[1]

Come back now to Ann Marie. She tells us that certain foods leave her exhausted, and that potato in particular sends her to sleep. Can we prove these assertions by skin or blood tests? Probably not. It would be highly unusual for IgE allergies to manifest themselves in this way. The truth is that we have very little understanding of the mechanisms by which these otherwise healthy foods have such an adverse effect on the health of susceptible individuals. So what are we to tell Ann Marie? Should we say that she is not allergic to these foods after all? Many reputable doctors would say just that! In relation to food, they reserve the term 'allergy' for type 1 (IgE) reactions alone, and refer to all other food reactions (including food aversion) as 'food intolerance'. Other doctors, equally clever, argue that von Pirquet's original concept of allergy was much broader than this, encompassing any state of 'altered reactivity', regardless of the mechanism. Perhaps you find yourself a victim of this awkward debate? Have you been told on the basis of negative skin and blood tests that you have no allergies, and yet still suspect that you react to certain foods? Read on.

Two schools of thought

As you can see, we have two conflicting schools of thought. The first relies heavily on objective tests and maintains that if we cannot show the *mechanism* of an allergy (by skin prick or blood test), then it's not an allergy. The contrasting view is empirical and much more comprehensive. It depends, not on theory, but on

1. Anaphylaxis is fully covered in *Could it be an Allergy?*

what we call clinical observation and experiment. If you get a symptom from an 'otherwise harmless' substance, you are (to put it simply) allergic to it. In this case, it does not matter whether we can understand the mechanism; it simply matters that we observe a symptom.

The strength of the first position is that it is built on 'hard science'; but herein also lies its weakness. As you can imagine, it is very reassuring to have a reliable test which gives objective evidence of an allergy. It makes the job a lot easier. However, we cannot dismiss a suspected allergy on the basis of our present inability to prove it in the laboratory. To do so would be to fall headlong into a scientific trap — a dark place where otherwise brilliant minds are restricted by the limitations of their machines. The purely scientific approach to allergy tests will lead to some patients being told that they are *not* allergic when, in fact, they *are*. Conversely, the broader proposition is founded on the art, rather than the science, of medicine. Once again, herein lie strength and weakness together. It is strong because it will consider greater possibilities. It will not dismiss what it cannot understand and, consequently, will not easily 'miss' an allergy. It is weak because it cannot always prove the truth of its own diagnosis, and because it is prone to all the variables of human nature. In particular, it is vulnerable to the placebo effect: a mysterious, beguiling and often potent human response to the power of suggestion. In this case, some patients will be told that they *are* allergic when, in fact, they are *not*.

Now I know this all sounds a bit academic, and please forgive me for that, but it does explain why there's so much confusion about. Personally, I have a great deal of sympathy with the former view, but I am also swayed by the everyday language of my patients. If they think they react to something, they tell me they're allergic to it, and they care not a wit whether I can understand it, measure it or explain it. Nevertheless, we must acknowledge the obvious difference that exists between these two kinds of allergy. One involves the immune system and causes inflammation; the other does not.

The fall-out

One of the dangers of strongly held opposing medical views is that we can lose sight of our patients in the process of argument. Many patients, who have become disillusioned with what they perceive as 'medical tunnel vision', have turned elsewhere for help. By virtue of its neglect, the medical profession has inadvertently flung the door open to the widespread use of quackery. Unqualified (and unregulated) persons have set themselves up as 'allergists', and have driven the allergy bandwagon rough-shod across every unexplained symptom. Innocent patients are told that they are allergic to various foods on the basis of unscientific and unreliable 'tests', such as vega machines, kinesiology, radionics etc. I know of one quack who can supposedly make a diagnosis over the phone: he asks the patient to hold a piece of hair against the telephone, and he swings his pendulum over the receiver at the other end of the line! It should come as no surprise to hear that patients are often given erroneous, and sometimes even dangerous, advice. 'But I had my allergies "tested" in such a manner,' you might say, 'and when I stopped eating certain foods I got better.' Fine. You stopped eating certain foods and you got better. In that case, you probably do have food intolerance, but the *method* of diagnosis is not thereby validated. To put it another way, I am not disputing the *diagnosis* of food intolerance in these cases, but I am most assuredly disputing the *methods* used to make the diagnosis. Patients who have their allergies tested in this way are usually told to avoid the following foods: wheat, dairy produce, eggs, yeast, and a few others like chocolate, coffee and citrus fruit. If everyone suspected of food intolerance were to avoid these foods, at least 25 per cent of them would get better. Why? Because these are the most commonly eaten foods in the European diet, and it is the most commonly eaten foods which most commonly cause allergic or intolerant symptoms. Americans, for instance, would have to add peanut and corn to this list (because they eat so much of them), and the Chinese, for the same reason, would need to pay more attention to rice and soy. To put an indefinite blanket exclusion on all these foods is usually unnecessary. The chances are that only one (or perhaps two) of these foods was causing symptoms, and that all the others are safe. With this in mind, patients invariably experiment to see what they can get away with; but because their food challenges are not properly conducted, they fail to accurately identify their culprit foods. Apart from the social nuisance of a restricted diet, there is also the danger of nutritional deficiency, and doctors have been left (on more than one occasion) to pick up the pieces of such disasters. Consider for a moment the true story of a frazzled mother who brought her hyperactive child to the doctor. 'Do you think it might be an allergy, doctor?' 'No chance! Here's an appointment for the behavioural therapist, and if that doesn't work, we'll give him some medicine to calm him down.' But the mother was not satisfied, so she took him away from the medics and into the hands of an unqualified person who told her (by magical means, and for a small fee) that the little chap was allergic to milk. She promptly excluded all dairy produce from his diet, and because she was not given adequate nutritional advice, he developed a bad case of rickets (a deficiency of vitamin D which seriously damages bone structure). She took him back to the doctor who was justifiably horrifed at the result. 'Didn't I tell you it wasn't an allergy? Now look what you've done!' The woman was thus further isolated from the profession, and the vicious cycle continues. The only beneficiaries in this scenario are the quacks. I must qualify two points. Firstly, not all hyperactivity is caused by food allergy, although more than half the cases are; and behavioural therapy, with or without medication, is an appropriate treatment for those which are not. Secondly, I do not wish to discredit 'alternative medicine'. Numerous patients have received lasting benefit from its practitioners, many of whom have had to pick up the pieces left behind by clumsy doctors! My plea — and this would be shared by genuine practitioners of alternative medicine — is that it be practised by persons qualified to do so, who understand all the issues involved in health care, and who are aware of the long-term consequences of their treatment regimes.

Case history

Carmel was a 48-year-old teacher. She had a miserable life, dogged by constant illness. The day she came to see me was a relatively good day, she explained, but she was plagued with symptoms even as she spoke. She was tired all the time, she had no energy, and she had one sore throat after another. 'I've even got one now', she protested, in obvious discomfort. She took a moment to massage her throat and continued with her story. 'My bowels are giving me gyp, and I have pains all over my body, and — ', she hesitated, as if she had suddenly remembered something. She just sat there for a while, gazing at the floor, her mouth still ajar in silent mid-sentence. Then, rather nervously, she raised an inquisitive eyebrow in my direction. No, I did not think she was mad, I reassured her, and I asked her to tell me more. It quickly became clear that Carmel had a multitude of symptoms, apparently unrelated. She had pains in her muscles and joints, her fingers and ankles were often swollen, she had mouth ulcers, bloating of the abdomen, constipation, abdominal pain, an itchy bottom, her sleep pattern was all over the place, her concentration was poor and her libido was low. Furthermore, her skin had 'gone to pot', especially just before a period. She had other premenstrual symptoms: her breasts were sore and she was particularly cranky for a week or so leading up to a period. As is so often the case, Carmel's previous investigations had drawn a blank, and she had been told that she was 'just depressed'. But Carmel would have none of it. 'Look,' she said, 'every time I eat wheat my throat flares up, and when I eat sugar I get depressed. What I want to know is could it be an allergy?'

Could it be an allergy?

Now there's a question that needs to be answered; for if Carmel does have an allergy, or several allergies, she could expect to find relief from her symptoms by avoiding the thing(s) she is allergic to. As with Ann Marie, Carmel's skin and blood tests were negative for allergy. However, it would be quite wrong to leave it there. As we've said, blood tests can only show IgE allergies; they do not reveal other kinds of allergy. This being the case, Carmel was put on the low allergy diet. She was advised to eat ten prescribed foods for a period of ten days. By the tenth day she felt better than she had done for years. All her symptoms without exception had disappeared. When she expanded her diet again, she reacted adversely to many of her staple foods. To cut a long story short, Carmel had multiple food intolerance.

Polysymptomatics

Carmel is not unusual. There are many like her who suffer for years on end with puzzling and debilitating symptoms. They have been on the merry-go-round of negative investigations, they have tried various medical treatments and, ultimately, they are at risk of being dismissed. Some of them are labelled neurotic or anxious; others are told they are depressed; and a few are said to be hypochondriacal. They can see the poorly disguised heart-sinking look on their doctor's face when they present with yet another baffling symptom, and another entry into the case notes sheaf which, at this stage, is as thick as a telephone directory. Many of them will give up going to their doctor altogether for fear they will be considered mad. The true nature of their illness lies buried in a jungle of *apparently* unrelated symptoms, and it lies there hidden for years until someone finally decides to look for it! It must be said that some of us *are* neurotic and anxious, and many of us *do* suffer from depression and/or hypochondriasis. We must also recognise that these disturbed mental states do give rise to physical symptoms. It is important therefore to keep an open mind in all this. But my plea is that psychiatric diagnoses should only be made in the presence of a positive history of psychiatric illness, and they should never be used to fob off symptoms that are otherwise difficult to resolve. The most common mistake in medicine is to assume that an illness is psychological when it isn't. The symptoms of food intolerance present a classical example of this.

Food intolerance

Food intolerance is far more common than food allergy. The principal difference between the two is timing (although this is not a hard and fast rule). We have already said that food allergy tends to show a rapid onset of symptoms; but in food intolerance there is a notable delay between the encounter with the offending food and the resulting symptom. Because of this delay, patients usually fail to recognise the relationship between what they eat and how they feel. There is a growing body of evidence to suggest that these 'hidden allergies' are responsible for many cases of migraine, irritable bowel syndrome, rhinitis, inflammatory bowel disease, arthritis, hyperactivity, chronic fatigue and others (see Table 4, page 138).

Unfortunately, we do not fully understand what happens in the body during delayed (non-IgE) reactions. However, we do have some idea of the mechanisms involved. Let us take a brief look at some of these.

1. Pharmacological activity of food

Some food reactions are the result of powerful natural substances present in food. These chemicals exert drug-like effects in our bodies. We refer to this phenomenon as 'false food allergy'. False, only because it looks like an allergy, but isn't. Here are a few examples.

Caffeine, an alkaloid drug. The most widely used foods with pharmacological activity are tea and coffee. An excessive consumption of caffeine may give rise to diverse toxic symptoms (see Chapter 16).

Histamine-containing foods. High levels of histamine occur naturally is some foods. This is a chemical we have already discussed at length in relation to allergic reactions. Histamine-containing foods include fermented cheeses and other foods, sausages, tinned foods (especially tinned smoked herring's eggs), sauerkraut and spinach. These foods, when eaten in excess and/or in combination, can cause:

- Flare up of eczema
- Headache
- Hot flushes
- Urticaria
- Angioedema
- Abdominal pain
- Thirst
- Shock (rarely)

Histamine-liberating foods. Some foods do not contain histamine, but they release histamine from mast cells in the body. This is a direct effect that does not involve IgE. Histamine-liberating foods include egg white, fish (especially shellfish), tomato, chocolate, pork, pineapple, strawberry, papaya and alcohol. They can also cause histamine symptoms.

Vasoactive amines. Vasoactive amines are also natural components of food. They have a drug-like effect on blood vessels (*vaso*), making them dilate. This gives rise to blood vessel headache (migraine). Histamine is one such amine. Others include phenylethylamine from chocolate (50 grams is enough to cause trouble), and tyramine in cheese, yeast extract, pickled herrings, bananas, broad beans, liver, sausage and alcohol.

Alcohol. Alcohol is an interesting food. Apart from its universal inebriating effect and its vasoactivity, it blocks enzyme pathways, has a diuretic effect, irritates the lining of the stomach and contains various food derivatives (and additives) to which some people are allergic.

2. Enzyme deficiencies

Food is digested by special enzymes in the gut, and further broken down by enzymes in the blood. Enzyme deficiencies will give rise to symptoms by allowing a build-up of particular food components in the gut or in the blood. One example that we should all be familiar with is our relative intolerance to onions. We don't have the enzyme necessary to digest the sugar in this food. High levels of sugar then reach the large intestine where they are fermented by resident microbes. Onions also contain a smelly disulphide. Excessive consumption of onions will therefore lead to smelly flatulence! Enzyme deficiencies may be more idiosyncratic, however. Lactose, for example, is the sugar found in milk. Some infants are born with a lactase deficiency, the enzyme by which we digest lactose. Lactose therefore builds up in the gut, causing a watery diarrhoea, and even collapse in some infants. Adults may acquire a transient lactase deficiency, especially after a bout of gastroenteritis, after intestinal surgery, or as a complication of another bowel disease. Milk consumption in such circumstances will also cause diarrhoea and related symptoms. Many other enzyme deficiencies have been identified, some of them causing serious health effects until they are diagnosed and treated by a lifetime of dietary avoidance. PKU (phenylketonuria) is probably the best known of these: every infant is checked for this at birth with the heel prick test.

3. Hormonal activity of foods

Food intolerance may also arise from foods that contain opium-like proteins. These include wheat, dairy produce and possibly corn. This may be linked to enzyme deficiency, for the proteins should be broken down by enzyme activity in the gut, and later in the blood. Symptoms known to be associated with opium-like proteins include mood and behaviour disorders, irritable bowel syndrome and water retention.

4. Toxins in food

It is hardly necessary to mention that some foods contain toxic chemicals that must be adequately degraded during cooking if they are not to cause trouble. Kidney (and other) beans, for example, should be soaked overnight and boiled for 90 minutes to break down the toxin therein. Abdominal cramps are the penalty for failing to take this precaution.

5. Sugars in food

Toddler's diarrhoea has been linked to the consumption of apple and other fruit juices. The mechanism here is, once again, fermentation of undigested and unabsorbed sugars in the large intestine. Other symptoms include abdominal discomfort, flatulence and borborygmi (those gurgles you hear coming from your bowels). Sugar malabsorption may also affect adults.

6. Other components of food

Vegetables, like fruit, contain indigestible sugars, such as raffinose, and may cause a similar fermentation reaction. They also contain other active components. Flavone compounds, for example, are known to affect intestinal motility. This leads to abdominal distension and discomfort in susceptible people. Cabbage is notorious in this regard. Another fairly common problem is fatty food intolerance. Fats are digested by bile from the gall bladder. They can cause a great deal of trouble for patients with gall bladder disease.

7. Unknown immune reactions

It must be said that the immune system does not sit idly by during all food intolerant reactions. Desensitisation for food intolerance is very effective and works by re-educating the immune system in some way (see Appendix 1). This suggests that food intolerance may involve the immune system after all. IgE and other antibodies are not involved, we know, but perhaps other immune mechanisms are. For example, a food may cause the release of immune chemicals not yet measured routinely in hospital laboratories. These chemicals have profound effects on the brain and hormone systems, and may thus easily give rise to symptoms. If this turns out to be the case, we shall have to redefine allergy yet again! The science of food intolerance is in its infancy, and we still have so much to learn. We have no simple clinical or laboratory test to help us in making a diagnosis (but see below). It is therefore hard to prove that a genuine reaction to food is actually taking place. Needless to say, if you are the one who has to endure a severe migraine headache or profound fatigue every time you eat a culprit food, you will not need convincing! But the sceptic will say: 'Might not the reaction be a psychological one?' And, of course, sometimes it is. There is a tendency for a small group of patients who are suffering from stress or depression to deny the true nature of their complaint, and to seek solace in what they consider to be the more socially acceptable and fashionable diagnosis of food allergy.

How do I find out if I have food intolerance?

The only reliable method for diagnosing food intolerance is the low allergy diet. This involves a wash-out phase, followed by the sequential reintroduction of foods. Ideally, this should only be done under the supervision of a medical doctor with a special interest in food allergy and intolerance. The dietary investigation will take approximately six weeks to complete and will demand your full commitment throughout this time. It is therefore imperative that you choose six consecutive weeks from your diary which are free of important social occasions. If you do succumb to forbidden culinary delights during the diet, you will undo all your hard work! I would like to emphasise that this is the only reliable way to determine whether foods are causing your symptoms or not. It will be a sound investment of time and effort, and it may allow you to join the ranks of the innumerable company of patients who have found lasting relief from their allergic fatigue.

Case histories

Before we get into the details of the diet, take some heart from these case histories. Carol was 65 years old when she came to see me, complaining of chronic fatigue. This had become particularly severe over the previous six months. In addition, she felt increasingly frustrated and depressed and suffered frequent headaches. She also had heartburn, mouth ulcers, an itchy scalp and an itchy bottom. Within seven days of starting a low allergy diet, all her symptoms disappeared. The dreadful fatigue had gone and she felt much better in herself. Upon subsequent food challenge she reacted only to yeast — a cloud of exhaustion came over her within a few hours of eating it. She had no other food reactions apart from this one. So, as long as she avoids yeast, she enjoys good health and has plenty of energy. Her fatigue is now a thing of the past. Carol was fortunate in that she only had one culprit food, but the matter is not always that simple. The case of young Jimmy was much more complex. He was 7 years old when his mother brought him to see me. His main problem was one of hyperactivity, but he was also constantly fatigued. Paradoxically, he felt exhausted but unable to rest. In fact, he could not sit still for one moment! He was almost always grumpy, and at times became quite aggressive. Needless to say, he was a handful. He also complained of daily headache, bellyache and diarrhoea; and as if this wasn't enough, his nose and eyes were constantly itching and watery.

His mother told me that he had been quite intolerant of milk as a baby, and this made her wonder whether he had any other, as yet unrecognised, food allergies. In order to answer this question, he was prescribed a low allergy diet, which he stuck to rigidly for seven days. At the end of this time, he and his mother had noticed an enormous improvement in his overall condition. 'We have a new boy on our hands!' she said with a big smile. Indeed, every single symptom without exception had disappeared. He was no longer hyperactive and his fatigue had given way to a sense of well-being. Subsequent food challenges showed him to be intolerant to milk (as suspected), but he also reacted to peanuts, corn, and foods in the brassica family — cabbage, broccoli, sprouts and cauliflower. As long as he avoids these foods, he remains well.

You will have noticed that both these patients had other symptoms apart from chronic fatigue. Far from being a coincidence, this is the very reason why their fatigue was thought to be related to food in the first place. Whenever fatigue is accompanied by other food-related symptoms, we should be alerted to the possibility that the fatigue itself may also be allergic in origin. Have a look at the Table of symptoms which may be caused by food intolerance.

Table 4. Symptoms which may have a food intolerance component

Brain	headache fatigue autism	migraine depression	hyperactivity epilepsy
Digestive tract	mouth ulcers constipation peptic ulcers anal itch	indigestion diarrhoea irritable bowel syndrome	nausea infantile colic Crohn's disease
Skin	eczema angioedema	urticaria bruising	itchy skin
Musculo-skeletal	muscle pains	arthritis	
Respiratory	asthma glue ear	sinusitis	rhinitis
Kidney and bladder	nephrotic syndrome	frequency of micturition	enuresis

Dietary investigation for food intolerance

Before embarking on the low allergy diet, take a note of your existing dietary habits. Studies have shown that dietary histories obtained by recall are notoriously unreliable, so a prospective seven day food dairy — in which you record everything that passes your lips — is advised. Apart from providing (i) the basis for accurate nutritional assessment, it will (ii) reveal whether you have cravings for any particular foods. Remember to include *everything*: main meals, snacks, biscuits, savouries, fruit, sweets, chocolate, tea, coffee, soft drinks, milk etc.

(I) NUTRITIONAL ASSESSMENT

A qualified dietitian is best placed to analyse your diet for its nutritional value (such detail is beyond the scope of this text). My concern here is that some patients put themselves on severely restricted and grossly inadequate diets. They do so to obtain relief from the unpleasant symptoms they experience from culprit foods. The problem for some is that, having excluded one or two offending foods, they become sensitised (intolerant) to the foods which they are now eating in greater quantity. Consequently, they exclude the 'new' offenders and restrict their diets even further. They have no choice now but to eat more and more of fewer and fewer safe foods. The tendency to sensitise does not abate, and they gradually exclude all but one or two food items. They falsely believe that they are not allergic to these few foods, but they may be. Allergic symptoms are not apparent, however, because the body is swamped with allergen and unable to respond. Such sensitive patients are, thankfully, rare. They need an expert allergist's help to get them out of the condition into which they have inadvertently placed themselves. One of the best ways out of this dilemma is a course of enzyme potentiated desensitisation (see Appendix). (A word of warning here: we must not be deceived by the young woman with *anorexia nervosa* who tries to disguise her eating disorder under a veil of 'multiple allergy'.)

(II) FOOD CRAVINGS

The food addict craves a particular food, and he feels unwell if he does not get a regular supply of it. He subconsciously gravitates towards the culprit food because he somehow knows that it will make him feel better. If he misses a dose, he will experience several withdrawal symptoms. Headache, muscle pain, fatigue and mood changes are common. Eating another dose will temporarily relieve his symptoms, but he has to increase his consumption to keep his symptoms at bay. He is on a slippery downward slope, and his health will gradually deteriorate over time. Thus, food cravings are frequently developed against a background of food intolerance/addiction and withdrawal.

Case histories

David came to see me recently at the age of 52. He told me about his long struggle with rhinitis, fatigue, low mood and anxiety. In addition, he suffered from weekly migraine headaches. His dietary history was informative. He had already discovered that yoghurt and cheese caused headache, so he avoids them now. However, he still drinks a lot of milk. He volunteered the fact that milk helps him to sleep — so much so that he cannot sleep without it. Furthermore, if he has to go without it for any length of time, he becomes restless, agitated and anxious. Drinking it again immediately relieves his feeling of tension. Drinking larger quantities actually depresses him and makes him feel fatigued, but he prefers to be depressed and fatigued than anxious and restless. You can see that he has the classical features of a food intolerance/addiction cycle. His intolerant symptoms are fatigue, depression and (probably) migraine. His withdrawal symptoms are restless agitation and anxiety. He will never enjoy good health as long as he remains in this vicious circle. He must stop consuming milk, and he must suffer the *transient* withdrawal symptoms of anxiety and restless agitation. These will give way, within a week or so, to a sense of well-being.

If you are craving a particular food, avoid it completely for seven to thirty days. In so doing, make sure you exclude it in all its different forms. For example, a dairy-free diet would have to exclude milk, skimmed milk, cream, ice cream, cheese, yoghurt, chocolate, whey, casein, caseinates, lactalbumin, lactose, and any processed food or recipe which contains these. You may find that this relatively simple step is sufficient to provide lasting relief from your symptoms.

The following case study, which was reported in the *British Medical Journal*, also illustrates the food intolerance/addiction phenomenon nicely. A 38-year-old mother of three presented with an eleven year history of severe and progressive rheumatoid arthritis. Every possible treatment known to doctors was tried, including steroids, anti-inflammatories, gold injections, immuno-suppressants etc. These not only failed to bring about relief, but caused her much additional discomfort in terms of adverse effects. One observant doctor noticed that she had a passion for cheese. Upon further enquiry he discovered that she consumed up to 1 lb of cheese per day, and had done so since her early twenties. He suggested that she try a dairy-free diet. Within three weeks she felt considerably better and she continued to improve over the following ten months (thus excluding a placebo effect). Her joints were no longer stiff, swollen or painful, her grossly abnormal blood tests reverted to normal and she no longer needed steroids. She suffers a relapse of arthritic symptoms within twelve hours of an accidental consumption of milk products.

Food craving and obesity

The foregoing discussion on the topic of food craving raises an inevitable question: are people who overeat doing so because of a hidden food allergy? The answer to this is yes, in a small minority of cases. One such woman was Noreen, a 40-year-old mother of two who came to see me with a life-long history of headaches. She also complained of rhinitis, sinusitis, generalised aches and pains, ankle swelling and obesity (she was three stone overweight). After a fourteen day wash-out period, during which she ate the low allergy diet, her symptoms were very much improved. She had no headache, her nose was dry, her ankles slim and she had lost a half-stone in weight (fluid loss). She continued to lose weight throughout the reintroduction phase. Not only did she identify the foods responsible for her headaches, but she also identified which foods gave her cravings for more food ('the crazy hungries', as she calls them). In her case these were wheat, sugar and soy. As long as she avoided these, she was able to lose weight 'effortlessly', and without craving. If she did eat them, on the other hand, she found herself on an uncontrollable binge. She lost three stone in as many months and she is virtually headache free.

Please note that Noreen was obese because she had eaten more energy than she had burned up, and the excess energy was stored as fat. She lost weight because she burned up more energy than she ate over time. Obesity is *not* an allergic disease; it's the result of eating too much. If food intolerance makes you crave, you are likely to eat more, and *that* is why you put on weight!

The low allergy diet (stage 1)

The first active step in dietary investigation is to rid the body of as many food allergens as possible. This 'wash-out' has two benefits. Firstly, symptoms that disappear may be considered intolerant in origin; and secondly, the body's reaction to the subsequent reintroduction of food allergens will be much more acute, thus enabling you to accurately identify culprit foods. Theoretically, the best wash-out of all is a total fast during which you drink only bottled or filtered water. This is a demanding task, however, and one which is not easily adhered to — especially by those who have domestic or employment duties. Fortunately, most patients do just as well by eating the low allergy diet. This consists of ten foods, or so, which we know from clinical experience to be of low allergy potential, i.e. they are the least likely to cause allergic problems. Remember that commercially available foods may be contaminated with chemicals such as pesticides, herbicides and fertilisers. These may cause symptoms in susceptible individuals. Organically grown produce is chemically free and therefore ideal for the low allergy diet. However, in practice most patients will do just as well on non-organic foods, but bear in mind that failure to obtain relief on this diet may be due to chemical sensitivity.

WITHDRAWAL SYMPTOMS

Many patients who go on this diet experience withdrawal symptoms. A headache often starts on the evening of the first day, or during the course of the second day. On days 2, 3 and 4, muscular pains similar to those that accompany the flu are prominent (but not invariable). Fatigue and low mood are also common features of the withdrawal phase. You can avoid the unpleasant combination of caffeine *and* food withdrawal symptoms occurring together by slowly reducing your caffeine intake over two weeks *before* starting the diet. Needless to say, it is possible to contract another illness by pure coincidence whilst on the diet; so if you are worried about the severity of your presumed withdrawal symptoms, have this checked out by your doctor. A word of caution follows for all patients with migraine, and for young boys with moderate or severe eczema.

Migraineurs

If you have ever lost your sight, or the power in a limb, or if you have ever had an epileptic fit during a migraine attack, you should *not* go on this diet without medical say-so. The danger is that you would suffer the worst migraine attack of your life, and there is a small risk that this could leave you with permanent neurological damage. There are other options for you, and these you should discuss with your clinical allergist.

Boys with moderate or severe eczema

As mentioned above, one of the benefits of a wash-out phase is that subsequent reactions to food challenges are much more acute. For some unknown reason, young boys with moderate or severe eczema may become *exquisitely* sensitive to the allergens in cow's milk after a wash-out period. The imprudent reintroduction of cow's milk may then precipitate a life-threatening reaction. The correct procedure for a milk challenge in such cases is for the doctor to rub a drop of milk on to the child's lip and wait for five minutes. If the lip does not swell, the child is given 5 ml of milk to drink. If there is no reaction within twenty minutes, the child is given a greater amount of milk, and so forth.

A typical low allergy diet starts off with the following (preferably fresh) foods:

- Lamb, salmon, cod, plaice
- Broccoli, parsnip, sweet potato (yams), turnip, courgette
- Kiwi, pears

- Use olive oil for cooking
- Drink only bottled spring water, natural (flat) or carbonated (fizzy).

The chances of inadvertently admitting a culprit food are reduced by further excluding all the foods on this list that you eat regularly, that is, more than once per week. If, for example, you eat a lot of lamb, substitute this with duck; similarly, try runner beans instead of turnip, chinese beansprouts for parsnip, rice for sweet potato, well-cooked cabbage for courgette, pineapple for pear and melon for kiwi fruit. The fewer foods you eat, the greater your chance of success.

During stage 1, remember:

- It may be preferable to conduct the diet under medical supervision.
- Stay on the diet for 7–14 days, depending on your symptoms. Rheumatoid arthritics, for example, would need to stay on the diet for 14 days (and sometimes longer). They should also avoid meat.
- If it's not on the list, you can't have it! As you see, no bread, no cake, no sauces, no cereals, no ice cream, no milk etc.
- You can eat any amount of allowed foods, in any combination, at any time.
- You will be bored, but don't go hungry.
- You need starch for energy — eat sweet potato at least three times per day.
- You should buy everything fresh. You can freeze it at home if you wish, because you won't add chemicals in the process.
- No smoking, no tea, no coffee.
- If you use salt, it should be pure sea salt without added chemicals.
- Use 1–2 teaspoons of Epsom salts for the first two days, especially if you are constipated, but not if you already have diarrhoea.
- Brush your teeth in bicarbonate of soda and water — toothpaste contains chemicals and corn. Put one teaspoon of bicarbonate into a glass of water, stir with your toothbrush and clean your teeth.

- Do not lick stamps or envelopes — the glue contains cornstarch and other foods.
- Check your medicines! Many drugs are packed in the factory with corn, potato, wheat, sugar etc. Avoid them if you can, but do not stop taking a prescribed drug without first consulting your doctor. It is dangerous to stop medication without advice.
- This is a diagnostic diet. It is therefore very important to stick *rigidly* to the allowed foods. This is the *only way* to find out if foods are causing your symptoms or not.
- You may feel worse in the first few days with headache, muscle pain, fatigue and low mood. These are withdrawal symptoms. They feel like the flu. If they are severe, take soluble paracetamol and a hot drink of bicarbonate of soda (2 tsp in hot water).
- It would be wise, while you're at it, to stay away from chemical exposures during this time. Remove all sources of chemicals, namely, anything that smells — bleach, pot-pourri, polish, perfumes, smelly soaps etc.

The low allergy diet (stage 2)

The low allergy diet will get rid of the symptoms of food intolerance. The very fact that symptoms disappear when you stop eating your regular foods is an indication that they were caused by those foods in the first place. Conversely, whatever symptoms you have left at the end of the diet cannot be blamed on the foods you haven't been eating. Therefore, if symptoms persist, abandon the investigation and seek expert help. The possibilities are

(i) You are not suffering from food intolerance, and your symptoms are due to something else entirely.
(ii) You are very unlucky to be intolerant to something allowed in the stage 1 diet.
(iii) Your symptoms are compounded by chemical sensitivity or gut fermentation.

You should only proceed to stage 2 if you have enjoyed a substantial reduction in symptoms. You are now in a position to test foods individually. The wash-out period of stage 1 accomplishes two things. Firstly, of course, it gets rid of your symptoms. Secondly, and just as important, it primes your system to react quickly to new foods as they are introduced. In other words, your intolerant reactions to a certain food will be much more obvious now because your system has had a good wash-out. Any departure from this state of relief must be considered a reaction until proven otherwise.

In stage 2 (and 3 and 4) we will try to bring your symptoms back! We will reintroduce foods one by one, and we will identify your culprit foods in the process. Most reactions to the foods on the list below will occur within five hours of ingestion, although some foods, such as the meats, may take a little longer. Longer reacting foods are tested in the evenings. This gives them the evening and the whole night to react (if they're going to). Thus, if you wake in the morning with a symptom, blame the new food from the night before. The golden rules are:

- New foods should be tested *one at a time*.
- Allow a five hour interval between each new food.
- Eat any safe food with the new food, or in between new foods.
- Any symptom experienced during testing must be blamed on the last new food introduced.
- Watch out for headache, joint pains, wheeze, runny nose, itchy skin, depression, fatigue, diarrhoea, bloating, nausea etc. Always blame the food — don't rationalise!
- If in doubt about a food, leave it out. It doesn't matter if a food is wrongly blamed because it can be easily retested (after a five day gap). It does matter if you unwittingly allow a culprit food to sneak back into your diet.
- If you get no reaction to a food, consider it safe and eat it as often as you like thereafter.
- If you get a reaction, stop testing new foods, and don't eat any more new foods until you are feeling well again. Continue to eat all your safe foods while you wait for the reaction to subside.
- If the reaction is severe, take soluble paracetamol and a hot drink of bicarbonate of soda (2 tsp in water)
- Reintroduce foods as follows:

Day	Breakfast	Lunch	Evening meal
1	Celery	Banana	Rice
2	Tomato	Carrots	Onion
3	Melon	Cauliflower	Beef
4	Tap water	Lettuce	Chicken
5	Oranges	Mushroom	Soybean[†]
6	Cow's milk (one glass)	Cabbage	Turkey
7	Tea (one cup only)	Apple	Yeast[¥]
8	Butter	Pineapple	Pork
9	Eggs	No new food*	Potato
10	Cheddar cheese	No new food*	Spinach

† Soak the beans for 8 hours, boil for 90 minutes, mash into minced beef and chopped onion (if safe) and make a burger.
¥ Crush three tablets of yeast into a safe food.
* Eggs and cheese may take longer than 5 hours to react.

Keep a detailed diary of foods eaten and symptoms experienced throughout the entire investigation:

New food tested	Time eaten	Symptoms, if any	List of safe foods
celery	Monday 8 a.m.	none	celery
banana	Monday 1 p.m.	headache after 30 minutes, lasted for 2 hours	–
rice	Monday 6 p.m.	none	rice

The low allergy diet (stage 3)

We now move on to cereals and sugars. These are different from

Day	New food	Notes
1 2 3	Wheat	Test in the form of wholemeal pasta, pure shredded wheat and/or home-made wholemeal bread — use wholemeal flour (no white flour added), bread soda, an egg (if safe) and buttermilk (if milk is safe). Some form of wheat must be eaten at each meal for the three full days.
4	Coffee Pepper	Fresh ground, one cup only for breakfast. Black peppercorn ground on evening meal.
5	Cane sugar	Demerara or muscovado (the brown one). Take 2 tsp at each meal for one full day.
6	Coconut Peanuts	Use dessicated or creamed, with breakfast. Use the raw ground (monkey) nut with the evening meal.
7	Beet sugar	Standard white table sugar. Take 2 tsp at each meal for 1 full day.
8 9	Corn	Use in two forms: corn on the cob and glucose powder. Also use home-made popcorn and pure cornflour if you like. Start each meal with fresh corn on the cob, and finish with 2 tsp of glucose powder.
10	Cauliflower Garlic	For breakfast. With the evening meal.
11 12	Oats	Test in the form of porridge, oatcakes and/or flapjacks (oat flake, safe sugar, butter). Eat some form of oats at each meal for two full days.
13	Malt	Use the extract, mix 2 tsp into a safe food at each meal for the full day.
14 15	Rye	Test in the form of Ryvita crispbread or pure rye bread. Eat some at each meal for two full days.

stage 2 foods, in that they do not always produce such an immediate reaction. They may take two or three days to produce symptoms. Thus, you could have wheat on Monday, Tuesday and Wednesday, and wake up on Thursday with a migraine. For this reason different rules apply, particularly in relation to the duration of each test. For the sake of variety, other foods are included here which will react within eight hours of ingestion.

N.B. Remember, if you wake up in the morning with symptoms, blame the last new food from the day before. Abandon a test as soon as you are sure that a reaction has occurred.

The low allergy diet (stage 4)

You now know which staple foods are safe and which ones cause you trouble. We now move on to stage 4. This is an open-ended stage, and it can go on as long as you like. During the first seven days we pay special attention to some of the chemicals added to food by man. Thereafter we test foods with multiple ingredients.

Day	New food	Notes
1	White bread	(Test only if wheat is safe.) This is a test for anticaking agents, bleaching agents etc.
2	Frozen peas	These are treated with sulphur dioxide and other chemicals.
3	Instant coffee	Roasted over an ethylene gas flame and contains many chemicals.
4	Tinned carrots	If you are safe with fresh carrots, but react to tinned carrots in water (phenolic resin lining the can), you will have to be careful with all tinned foods.
5	Monosodium glutamate	This is used as a flavour enhancer, especially in Chinese food.
6	Saccharin	A sweetener hidden in some soft drinks and confectionery. Take two tablets as a test.
7	Raisins	Also treated with sulphur dioxide.

You can now proceed to foods with multiple ingredients. This includes jams, sauces, chocolate, cake and biscuits etc. However, don't forget all the other possibilities: cucumber, grapefruit, dates, asparagus, lemon, lentils, prawns, sprouts, chick peas, almonds, herring, sunflower seeds etc. If you get a reaction from a food with multiple ingredients, you should be able to trace the source of your trouble (because you know your status with the main ingredients).

Is there a short cut?

I mentioned earlier that the foods most commonly eaten are the most likely to cause trouble. Wheat, dairy, sugars, yeast, corn, and the like, are among the most frequent offenders. It therefore stands to reason that a diet which excludes these (and only these) could have the same benefit as the 'gold-standard' low allergy diet. So if you are a bit daunted by the prospects of the latter, you could try the following diet for two weeks. We call it the 'hunter-gatherer' or 'stone age' diet. As the name suggests, it allows foods which you could have caught or collected on one of your outings from your 'cave' home.

For two weeks, eat *only*

- Fresh fruit   all kinds, with the possible exception of citrus fruit.
- Fresh vegetables   all kinds, with the possible exception of potato.
- Fresh meats   all kinds, not forgetting rabbit, venison, etc.
- Fresh poultry   all kinds, not forgetting duck, pheasant, quail, etc.
- Fresh fish   all kinds, including shellfish.
- Fresh nuts   all kinds, but must be fresh.
- Olive oil   for cooking.
- Sea salt   with no additives or preservatives.
- Drinks: bottled spring (or filtered) water, flat or fizzy, herbal teas.
  fruit juice prepared from your own fruit.

This diet excludes most tinned and packet foods
dairy produce and eggs
breads and other cereals
sugars, yeast and alcohol
tea and coffee.

For this diet to be successful, you must stick to the foods listed. If you are not sure whether a particular food is allowed, simply ask yourself if it falls into the main categories above. If it is a fruit or vegetable, it is allowed; if not, leave it out. So what about something like sweetcorn? Should that be allowed? No, corn is a cereal, not a vegetable! What about vinegar? No. Mustard? No. Monkey nuts? Yes. Avocado pear? Yes. And so forth.

If your symptoms clear within two weeks on this diet, well and good. You may now proceed to reintroduce the omitted foods as detailed above. If symptoms persist, then you will have no choice but to step down to the stricter low allergy diet. Please do not stay on this (or any other) diet for long periods without the benefit of expert nutritional advice.

Trouble-shooting

This is for patients who enjoy great relief from symptoms on the low allergy or stone age diets, and then get confused during the reintroduction phase. Your symptoms may have recurred without clear-cut reactions. In the first place, let me say this: never lose sight of the fact that you have food intolerance. Get expert help if you cannot figure out your culprit foods. There are several sources of confusion:

1. *You have allowed a culprit food to sneak into your diet.* Go back to the point where you last felt well and eat only those foods which you are sure of. Stay there for a few days until the symptoms clear again. Retest the foods, but this time *take larger portions.*
2. *Your reactions take longer than five hours.* Go back to the point where you last felt well and eat only those foods which you are sure of. Stay there for a few days until the symptoms clear again. Retest the foods, but this time *give them more time to react.* For example, allow one full day per stage 2 food; test wheat over one full week etc.

151

3. *You have gut fermentation.* In this case the symptoms will slowly return with a build-up of carbohydrate (starch and sugar) foods. Have a gut fermentation test (see below).
4. *You're drinking too much caffeine.* You had no reaction to one cup of tea (or coffee), you correctly thought you were not intolerant, and you started to drink too much of it. Stick to one cup of tea and one cup of coffee per day until the investigation is complete. Increase your consumption thereafter if you wish.
5. *Chemicals are accumulating.* The symptoms may result from the accumulation of natural and/or added chemicals as you expand your diet.

Dietary investigation complete. Now what?

You have now completed your dietary investigation for food intolerance. You have two options:

1. You can avoid your culprit foods. You may find that you can tolerate small amounts of your culprit foods after a prolonged period of abstinence, say six to twelve months. See what you can get away with!
2. You can opt for a course of enzyme potentiated desensitisation (see Appendix 1). This will increase your tolerance to culprit foods and allow you to eat them without feeling ill. If you have had multiple reactions, or if your culprit foods are hard to avoid socially and nutritionally, you should give this treatment serious consideration.

Meanwhile

- Try to vary the diet as much as possible. This will help to prevent the development of new allergies.
- Regular vigorous exercise is beneficial to the body in general, and to the immune system in particular.
- Beware of food cravings — they signal the emergence of new intolerance.
- Pay attention to your nutritional status — you need adequate supplies of all essential nutrients.

16 *Caffeine*

Caffeine is a drug. It belongs to the alkaloid family. Other members of the same family include morphine, cocaine, quinine, strychnine, nicotine and atropine. All these are used, or abused, in some way by man. Quinine and atropine are prescribed for certain medical conditions; morphine and cocaine are effective painkillers, and are widely abused by drug addicts; strychnine is a highly toxic poison; and nicotine is the well-known addictive substance in tobacco. Alkaloids are naturally occurring and are found in many plants. They are neurotoxins (nerve poisons) and their presence in plants is thought to protect them from being eaten by insects. Let me put it like this: an insect who feeds off a plant containing poisonous alkaloids may never eat again!

Caffeine is found (i) in the beans of the *Coffea* species, from which we make coffee; (ii) in the leaves of *Camellia sinensis*, from which we make tea; (iii) in the kola nut, which we use in cola drinks; (iv) in the cocoa bean, from which we make chocolate; and (v) in many pharmaceutical products such as cold remedies etc.

Caffeine-containing drinks are a relatively recent addition to the Western diet. Although tea has been used in China from as early as 2737 B.C., it was not brought to Europe until A.D. 1610, or to England until A.D. 1657. Similarly, coffee was first used in Arabia in the fourteenth century, but did not come to Europe until 300 years later. When it finally did, it was greeted with disdain and was greatly resisted by some. It was thought to be an intoxicating drink and one which was hazardous to health. It eventually became a socially acceptable drink, and it is now so widely used that researchers have difficulty in finding non-caffeine drinkers for comparison studies!

Symptoms caused by caffeine

Like most drugs, caffeine can be thought of as having desired effects, adverse effects and toxic effects. Like most alkaloids, caffeine is potentially addictive, in that we can develop tolerance (become immune to it) with regular usage, and suffer withdrawal symptoms when deprived of it.

The desired effect of caffeine (the reason we drink it in the first place) is mental stimulation. Studies on healthy volunteers suggest that the stimulant effect of caffeine helps to counteract fatigue in the short term. However, this is of limited value. It is very easy to take too much and to slip into a cycle of toxicity, tolerance and withdrawal, thus negating any beneficial effects.

Caffeine toxicity and tolerance

Susceptible individuals may experience toxic effects from as little as 100 mg of caffeine per day — that's just one cup of tea! Most of us, however, would tolerate 250 mg/day (three cups of coffee) before the onset of toxicity. The earliest symptoms of caffeine excess include:

- anxiety and restlessness
- excitement
- insomnia
- headache
- flushing of the face
- needing to pass water frequently
- tummy upsets (such as abdominal pain and diarrhoea).

Caffeine-induced anxiety can be severe; so much so that it has earned its own place in medical language — it is known as caffeinism. As previously discussed, anxiety may lead to hyperventilation, thus adding all the symptoms of that disorder to the already numerous symptoms of caffeinism.

Most readers will be aware of the propensity for caffeine to cause insomnia. This may occur as part of caffeinism, or it may be the only symptom you experience. Insomnia will, of course, give rise to all the consequences of chronic sleep deprivation, including chronic fatigue. The restless legs syndrome (previously discussed on page 91) is another caffeine-related disorder. Briefly stated, this is experienced as a feeling of extreme annoyance in the legs, especially severe at night in bed, and which can only be momentarily relieved by moving the legs. Often the legs move involuntarily — with sudden and violent jerks — and jolt the unfortunate sufferer out of the sleep for which he had waited so long. The end result is the prevention of restorative sleep. Anyone who has restless legs should give up caffeine, at least for a while, to see if it is contributing to the problem.

Higher doses of caffeine may give rise to other symptoms. For example, a single dose of 700 mg of caffeine (six cups of brewed coffee in quick succession) can push a healthy person into a classical panic attack, even if they have never had one before. The regular consumption of one gram per day can result in muscle twitching, ringing in the ears (tinnitus), flashing lights, rambling thought, incoherent speech, palpitations, agitation and episodes of inexhaustibility.

Very high doses of caffeine can be extremely dangerous. For instance, 10 grams as a single dose has been known to induce psychotic states in the previously healthy, and relapses in schizophrenics. These extraordinary doses may also cause convulsions, respiratory failure and death!

Chronic caffeine usage has also been implicated in certain cases of high blood pressure, worsening of the premenstrual syndrome and increased urinary and faecal loss of calcium — the latter having obvious relevance to the development of osteoporosis and the formation of kidney stones. Finally, there is a suggestion that excessive coffee intake over time (nine cups or more per day) is associated with an increased risk of death from heart disease in middle-aged men.

It must be said that the vast majority of caffeine drinkers develop a degree of tolerance to the drug. This allows them to drink regular doses without being aware of fluctuating symptoms. However, even these may experience toxic effects following a sudden increase, and withdrawal effects from a sudden decrease in consumption.

Caffeine addiction and withdrawal

'Now hold on a minute,' you may say, 'I feel much better after my cup of coffee [or tea], so how can you say it's bad for me? It wakes me up.' Ah yes, it wakes you up, but only because you were suffering from caffeine-withdrawal symptoms in the first place. For most habitual users, the feeling of stimulation is nothing more than the relief of withdrawal symptoms (which they wouldn't have if they didn't drink caffeine). Because it is addictive, any attempt to come off the drug will result in a recognised withdrawal reaction. Admittedly, withdrawal symptoms are more common in heavy caffeine users (500 mg/day or more), but they may also occur at the much lower level of 100 mg/day. Symptoms start within twelve hours of a missed dose, peak between twenty-four and forty-eight hours, and last for a week. The most common symptom is headache, but this may be accompanied by

- marked fatigue, and/or
- depression and anxiety, and/or
- nausea and vomiting, and/or
- we may become irritable and unfriendly.

Caffeine, when taken in a hot drink, is absorbed into the body within thirty-five minutes. This ensures a rapid top-up of blood levels and a rapid suppression of withdrawal symptoms. In other words, one cup of tea or coffee will quickly help the addict to feel better. This explains why some people just don't feel right until they have had their first dose of caffeine in the morning, and why they cannot function throughout the day unless they have a regular supply of it. It also explains the headache which some people get when they sleep in at the weekend. They are used to regular early morning doses of caffeine during working days, and they begin to suffer withdrawal symptoms when they don't get up early enough to top-up their levels on Saturday and Sunday mornings.

It is interesting to note that caffeine is eliminated from the body relatively quickly — within four to six hours — and that this rate of elimination is increased to less than two hours in those who smoke. Smokers will therefore need more regular cups of coffee to maintain their blood levels of caffeine. The problem is, they usually have a smoke with their drink! You can keep withdrawal symptoms to a minimum by slowly reducing your caffeine intake over two weeks. It is best to keep a diary and allow yourself a certain number of cups of your favourite drink per day until you have cut it out altogether, e.g., 25 cups today, 24 tomorrow, 23 the day after, and so on.

So how much caffeine is safe?

The average daily consumption of caffeine in Europe is approximately 400 mg per day. This gives an average blood level of 2 mg/l, which is certainly enough to cause symptoms in those more susceptible. Opinion is divided as to what a safe consumption of caffeine would be: some say 500 mg per day, but others reckon 250 mg (and that means only two cups of coffee or three cups of tea per day). Apart from the immediate symptoms of toxicity and withdrawal, there is a question mark over caffeine in relation to blood pressure and heart disease. Further research into this area is ongoing.

In any case, it is important to realise that some people are very sensitive to the pharmacological effects of caffeine, and their tolerance will be much lower than expected. These people will not feel well if they take any amount of caffeine, and the only realistic option for them is total abstinence. Patients with generalised anxiety can induce a panic attack with as little as one cup of coffee!

Children are also sensitive to caffeine, and particularly to its effects on the brain. They respond by exhibiting hyperactive behaviour, even to small doses, and for this reason they are often forbidden to drink tea or coffee. But cola drinks also contain significant amounts of caffeine. These are often overlooked, and seldom forbidden!

How to calculate your caffeine intake

It is important to make an accurate assessment of your daily consumption of caffeine. Go through a typical day in your mind's eye, and count each drink you have from the moment you wake up. Use the following values to calculate your total amount.

Remember that one mug is equal to 2 cups, so double your score if you drink mugs instead of cups.

Caffeine content of various drinks

Ground coffee	125–140 mg	per 225 ml cup
Instant coffee	70–100 mg	per 225 ml cup
Tea	60–100 mg	per 225 ml cup
Cola drinks	40 mg	per 330 ml can
Chocolate drinks	5 mg	per 225 ml cup

Well, how did you fare? Are you drinking more than 250 mg per day? It is not unusual to come across patients who ingest three grams of caffeine per day in the form of thirty cups of strong tea, or the equivalent! No wonder they complain of sleeplessness, nausea, agitation, fatigue, lethargy and so on. I usually recommend to anyone with chronic fatigue that they reduce their caffeine intake to nil, at least for a while. The same applies to anyone with a chronic anxiety state — *all* their symptoms may be due to the drug-like effects of caffeine. The tragedy is that such patients are not advised along these lines, and they end up taking tranquillisers, which in turn may add to their fatigue and lower their mood. These drugs may even worsen the symptoms of anxiety in some patients. Some people invest considerable time and effort in psychotherapy, looking for hidden reasons for their anxiety, whilst all the time their symptoms are caused by caffeine. It is ironic to imagine the anxious patient pondering over the possible significance of past life events as the psychologist scratches his head in puzzlement. 'Never mind love. Here, have another up of coffee!' (Alcohol has a similar anxiety-producing effect in some sensitive individuals, even when taken in small amounts.)

What about decaffeinated drinks?

I am often asked whether decaffeinated drinks are an acceptable substitute for the fatigued. The answer is: they are not, at least not initially. The problem is that coffee, for example, contains at least another 300 compounds besides caffeine; and although these have not yet been fully assessed, we know for sure that decaffeinated coffee is still capable of causing gastric symptoms in susceptible people. Similarly, tea contains other potentially harmful substances, including tannic acid. This acid is a potent inhibitor of iron absorption, and it may therefore lead to anaemia, which in turn will produce its own symptoms. Once you recover from your fatigue, you could drink tea and coffee again; but start with modest doses and keep an eye out for a return of old symptoms. You will need to keep your regular consumption below the symptom threshold.

17 Hypoglycaemia — Low Blood Sugar

Hypoglycaemia means low (*hypo*) blood glucose (*glycaemia*). Glucose is the single most important source of energy for the body, and whereas some cells are able to utilise substitute fuels under certain conditions, there are other cells which depend exclusively on glucose for their energy. They cannot function well unless they are provided with an adequate and steady supply of it. Chief among these are the brain cells (the retina in the eye and the reproductive cells are also glucose dependent). If the blood glucose level falls too low, the brain will suffer an 'energy crisis', and this will result in a number of mental as well as physical symptoms — not the least of which is fatigue.

More about glucose

Glucose, in biochemical terms, is a saccharide, i.e. a sugar unit. Because it is a single unit, it is called a monosaccharide. Fructose and galactose are examples of other monosaccharides. Some sugars consist of two monosaccharide units bound together, and these are known as disaccharides. Lastly, there are sugars which consist of very long chains of monosaccharide units bound together, and these are known as polysaccharides. Mono and disaccharides are simple sugars, whereas polysaccharides are complex. The relevance of these different sugars to hypoglycaemia will become clear shortly. Sugars are also called carbohydrates, so there is plenty of room for confusion over the terminology. In practice, these terms are used interchangeably.

Where does glucose come from?

In Chapter 12 we saw the importance of carbohydrate foods in relation to our health and well-being, with particular reference to glucose. Let us briefly recap on the biochemistry. There are three major sources of glucose in the normal human diet. These are:

- sucrose, which is the disaccharide sugar we buy in bags (consisting of glucose and fructose).
- lactose, which is the disaccharide sugar found in milk (consisting of glucose and galactose).
- starch, which is the polysaccharide sugar (consisting predominantly of glucose) found in almost all foods, but especially in the grains.

When these sugars are eaten, they are digested in the gut like any other food. The polysaccharides, being complex sugar molecules, are gradually broken down to their constituent monosaccharide units. Because each monosaccharide is bound to the next one in the chain, it takes a relatively long time to digest the whole polysaccharide. This ensures a gradual absorption of sugar into the blood. The disaccharides, on the other hand, need very little digesting because they only have one bond to be broken before releasing their two monosaccharide units. Finally, when sugar is ingested in the monosaccharide form, it needs no digestion at all. Ingestion of mono or disaccharide sugars will cause a rapid increase in blood glucose. This is where the concept of the glycaemic index comes from. Foods which give a rapid rise in glucose are said to have a high glycaemic index.

Glucose is by far the most important monosaccharide, so we can forget about the others and concentrate on it alone. It is more or less immediately absorbed into the blood and taken to the liver for processing. The liver, which has a large storage capacity, will hold on to about two-thirds of all the glucose ingested and, in doing so, will prevent the unacceptable rise in blood glucose levels which would otherwise occur after meals.

The remaining one-third passes directly into the blood and stimulates the pancreas to release insulin. Insulin then promotes the transport of glucose into the billions of cells around the body, thus providing them with essential energy, but causing a fall in blood glucose levels in the process. The liver detects the falling level of glucose and responds to it by releasing more of the glucose which it is holding on to, thus restoring the blood level to normal.

Normal blood glucose levels

In health, the level of glucose in the blood at any one time is carefully maintained within a specific and fairly narrow range. This is achieved by the balanced interaction of: (a) the two pancreatic hormones, insulin and glucagon; (b) the liver; and (c) the stress hormone adrenaline. The pancreas, of course, is better known for the enzymes it secretes into the intestine for the digestion of food, but it also contains two other cell types — one which secretes insulin, and the other which secretes glucagon directly into the blood. There are also mechanisms in place to increase the availability of glucose when levels are low. Firstly, the brain stimulates the adrenal glands to release adrenaline. Adrenaline, in turn, will stimulate the liver to release glucose into the blood (this action of adrenaline makes perfect sense: it provides a rapid increase of blood glucose to facilitate the fight or flight response for which it is usually secreted in the first place). Secondly, the pancreas will secrete glucagon, which also stimulates glucose release from the liver, and indeed it is far more effective than adrenaline in this respect. Thus glucose levels are maintained within a very specific range. This ensures firstly a steady supply of energy to glucose-dependent cells; and secondly that glucose levels are not allowed to rise to potentially dangerous heights. (Diabetes mellitus is a condition in which glucose levels are too high (*hyper*glycaemia).

How do we define hypoglycaemia?

Actually there are two types of hypoglycaemia to consider. One is called 'spontaneous', the other 'reactive' (or functional). The definition of spontaneous hypoglycaemia is a biochemical one. We can measure the blood glucose level directly, and because we know what the normal range is, we can easily and objectively tell whether it is too low or too high. The (arterial) blood glucose level must fall to at least 3.0 mmol/l before symptoms of hypoglycaemia are experienced, and even then the symptoms will be very mild. More noticeable symptoms occur when levels fall below 2.2 mmol/l. Age plays a part in this variability, so we define hypoglycaemia as an arterial blood glucose level lower than 2.2 mmol/l in subjects younger than 60 years, and lower than 3.0 mmol/l in those aged 61 years or older. This is an arbitrary definition — symptoms may occur above these levels (especially in diabetics) and do not necessarily occur below them. There is no controversy in medical circles about the definition, diagnosis or treatment of spontaneous hypoglycaemia.

Reactive hypoglycaemia is more difficult to define because it cannot be measured in the laboratory. Once again we find ourselves facing two opposing schools of medical thought. And that's a pity because reactive hypoglycaemia is of great interest to us in relation to fatigue. We'll come back to this later, but let us first understand the spontaneous variety.

Spontaneous hypoglycaemia

Symptoms of hypoglycaemia are the direct result of falling levels of glucose in the brain. This is called neuroglycopenia, and it may occur in several recognised phases: acute (short time frame), subacute (medium time frame) and chronic (longer time frame).

Acute symptoms are those which arise when the levels of glucose first begin to fall. They include general feelings of malaise, anxiety and panic, palpitations, blurred vision and trembling. These will be well known to diabetics as the first symptoms of an impending 'hypo'. In fact, diabetics are experts on hypoglycaemia, and we have learned a lot of what we know about this subject from them. They must be careful not to overdose themselves with insulin into a hypoglycaemic state. As mentioned above, insulin reduces the blood sugar to normal by promoting the transport of glucose into cells. Too much insulin will cause too much glucose to enter the cells, and the blood level will fall dramatically. Sometimes the fall can be so profound as to plunge the patient into a coma. This is a medical emergency requiring the immediate injection of intravenous glucose and/or glucagon (which will rapidly mobilise glucose from the liver into the blood).

Subacute symptoms creep up on you gradually over time: a general slowing down, a loss of spontaneous movement and activity, mental dullness and sleepiness. If untreated, this too could progress to coma.

Chronic symptoms are very rare and result from long-term low glucose levels. This can be achieved only by insulin-secreting tumours or the excessive use of insulin over weeks or months. The net effect is nerve damage in the brain. Symptoms include depression (which may be severe), schizophrenic thought and behaviour, and dementia.

Causes of spontaneous hypoglycaemia

A number of rare medical conditions are known to induce spontaneous hypoglycaemia. These include:

- the excessive insulin production of a pancreatic tumour (which causes a huge shift of glucose out of the bloodstream and into the cells).
- certain cancers (which utilise vast quantities of glucose at the expense of other cells).
- liver disease (in which the liver is unable to respond to falling levels of glucose).
- the hypoglycaemia which follows certain abdominal operations.

Reactive hypoglycaemia

The concept of reactive hypoglycaemia is a controversial one. It was first proposed as an explanation for the clinical observation that some patients with symptoms of hypoglycaemia did not, in fact, have low blood glucose levels. In other words, they complained of low blood sugar symptoms, even though their blood sugar levels were normal. The suggestion is that these patients experience symptoms when their blood glucose levels are *falling*, not just when they are below our arbitrary figures of 3.0 or 2.2 mmol/l. In these cases it is the *rate* of fall that is thought to be important, not the actual level.

The typical presentation is a patient who complains of anxiety, nervousness and sweating, headache, irritability and feelings of faint. These symptoms come on several hours after a meal and can be relieved by sugar. Sometimes these patients feel perfectly well in between attacks, but more commonly they complain of chronic fatigue. This is why the concept of reactive hypoglycaemia is of interest to those who are fatigued. In fairness to science, it may be better to refer to this as the postprandial (after-a-meal) syndrome, because we are not convinced of the precise mechanisms involved.

As I've said, it may be that they are sensitive to the rate of glucose fall, and their brain responds too readily by stimulating the adrenal glands. This would represent the brain's attempt to release glucose from the liver and thus restore blood levels to normal. However, adrenaline is a stress hormone, and whenever there is a surge of adrenaline release, symptoms of the fight or flight response are produced, namely, increased heart rate, irritability, aggression, sweating, anxiety and nervousness.

Some of these patients also report a craving for sugars and an inability to miss out on meals. They have discovered that their symptoms will disappear if they eat something sweet. Although this will help them to feel better, it will only be for a short time. In the long term, the patient becomes a sugar addict, craving for sweet things — 'Anything, so long as it's sweet.' The sugar they eat will of itself cause an excessive rise in glucose levels, and this will inevitably be followed by another drop. Sugar levels may thus swing from peak to trough throughout the day in an endless and uncontrolled cycle. The patient never feels well. She resorts to sugar-laden snack after snack in order to pull herself through the day. She doesn't know it, but although she is constantly trying to increase her sugar (and energy) level, she is only aggravating her condition by doing so.

Can sugar cause reactive hypoglycaemia?

When modest amounts of sugar are eaten in their natural form (whole fruit, vegetables and grain), they are gradually broken down in the intestine and gradually absorbed into the blood. These foods have a low glycaemic index. The liver and pancreas have plenty of time to process the glucose and blood levels are kept well within the normal range. Hypoglycaemia does not arise in this situation.

In contrast, foods with a high glycaemic index (e.g. refined sugars) may cause trouble in susceptible individuals. Rapid increases in blood glucose may quickly saturate the liver storage capacity, allowing glucose to 'spill over' into the bloodstream. The pancreas responds urgently by secreting large amounts of insulin in a desperate bid to bring the situation back under control. Blood glucose levels then fall precipitously, and possibly to very low levels. Symptoms of the postprandial syndrome and/or hypoglycaemia ensue. Thus reactive hypoglycaemia may occur as an *over-reaction* to the ingestion of large amounts of sugar.

Factors aggravating reactive hypoglycaemia

(1) STRESS

The stress hormone adrenaline exerts an effect on the liver, causing an increase in blood sugar levels. This increase is appropriate when sugar levels are low, or when some strenuous exercise is anticipated. But patients who are experiencing stressful life circumstances, whether real or perceived, will secrete excessive amounts of adrenaline into their blood. This produces the well-known physical symptoms of anxiety, namely, rapid heart rate, palpitations, dry mouth, dilated pupils, sweating, diarrhoea, frequency of micturition and headache. The excessive adrenaline released in this situation will cause an inappropriate elevation of glucose, thereby adding to the already unstable swings in blood glucose levels.

(2) PERSONALITY

Some authorities have suggested that there are particular personality traits associated with reactive hypoglycaemia. Needless to say, these are seldom flattering! Doctors suffer from a seemingly irresistible urge to pigeon-hole their patients into clearly defined boxes. I suggest that you take the description of the hypoglycaemic personality with a judicious amount of salt, and allow yourself a wry smile! Hypoglycaemic individuals are supposed to be 'thin, tense, hyperkinetic young women' who are of a 'compulsive, conscientious and intense personality'. I mention this because we must remember that hypoglycaemia can itself produce personality changes. Correcting this may result in a significantly different person, having more energy, a clearer mind and being considerably less anxious. Furthermore, the ability to concentrate and to memorise may also improve, and those who are prone to disturbed thought will also notice a quietness of mind.

(3) ALCOHOL, CAFFEINE, AND NICOTINE

Alcohol, caffeine and nicotine, all of which interfere with the body's ability to handle sugar, can aggravate hypoglycaemia. Smoking initially stimulates the pancreas to secrete glucagon, producing an increase in blood glucose levels, but this is followed by insulin secretion, which results in hypoglycaemia. The widespread habit of turning to sweet foods when trying to give up cigarettes may be a subconscious attempt to increase blood sugar levels. The nicotine isn't there to stimulate glucagon secretion, so the sugar level has to be increased in some other way. It is actually easier to give up smoking whilst on a hypoglycaemic diet.

Patients who are prone to hypoglycaemia should not drink alcohol with their meals. They would likewise be well advised to decline the offer of finishing their meal with coffee and/or a smoke. Whereas some individuals would seem to get away with such an occasional splurge, the hypoglycaemic will not.

(4) NUTRITIONAL DEFICIENCY

Certain nutritional factors are essential to the body's ability to handle glucose. One of these is the trace element chromium. Without it, insulin is not as effective in transporting glucose to the cells. In fact, chromium has been called 'glucose tolerance factor', and it is being investigated as a possible adjunct in the treatment of diabetes. Supplementation with chromium may also be helpful to non-diabetics, but only if a true deficiency exists. This can only be determined by a sophisticated laboratory investigation. If chromium supplements are taken in the absence of a true deficiency, toxic effects such as disturbed sleep pattern, vivid and frightening dreams and increased irritability may be produced. Brewer's yeast is a good natural source of chromium. A number of other essential nutrients are required for glucose handling. These include manganese, magnesium and the B vitamins, to name but a few.

(5) PREMENSTRUAL SYNDROME

Women often report a craving for sweet things in the days or weeks leading up to their menstrual period. Many also complain of increased appetite, fatigue, dizziness and faintness as part of their premenstrual syndrome. These are similar to the symptoms of hypoglycaemia. The hormonal changes of the menstrual cycle make some women more prone to hypoglycaemia at this time. The contraceptive pill may occasionally cause similar problems.

Treatment of hypoglycaemia

The symptoms of spontaneous hypoglycaemia will respond rapidly to the ingestion or injection of sugar. Injections of glucagon are also very useful in these situations. The symptoms of reactive hypoglycaemia (or postprandial syndrome) can also be reversed by sugar in the short term. However, better and sustained results can be achieved by adopting the following dietary pattern. Remember that carbohydrates should constitute 70 per cent of our energy intake. So we are not condemning sugar *per se*. The main change has to do with the timing of meals, not their meal content.

- Exclude all the highly refined carbohydrates such as biscuits, jams, cake, chocolate, sweets, honey and puddings. In practice, this means avoiding many processed foods, as most of these have added sugar. Read the labels and watch out for such sugars as glucose syrup, corn syrup, maltose, dextrose, dextrin, maltodextrin, lactose, and so forth. Obviously, spoonfuls of sugar are not allowed, even if they are supposed to 'help the medicine go down'! Certain medicines are laced with sugar, and these should be substituted for healthier equivalents, if possible.
- Wholemeal bread, potato and rice are good sources of carbohydrate. They have a low glycaemic index.
- Eat six small meals a day. This will ensure that large amounts of carbohydrate do not get into the system all at once, and the blood sugar level should be more stable as a consequence.
- Eat more fruit and vegetables, eggs, cheese, fish, meat and nuts.
- As well as six small meals per day, take some form of snack every two hours. This should consist of fruit, fruit juice, nuts, cheese etc.
- Avoid factors that are known to aggravate hypoglycaemia: alcohol, caffeine and nicotine.

• Remember that the adrenaline released in times of tension or anxiety will produce physical symptoms of its own, as well as aggravating the problem of hypoglycaemia. Furthermore, it may also complicate the hyperventilation syndrome, as pointed out in a previous chapter. If you experience difficulty in handling stress, whether real or perceived, it may be that you would derive some benefit from expert counselling in this area.

Case history

Lara is an active person. Not only does she maintain a busy study schedule in a technical college, but she runs a local cultural centre as well. It is not unusual for her to put in a twelve hour day at the centre, and then return home to start studying! Her weekends are taken up with fund-raising activities, without which the centre would probably have to close. She is 23 years old, and has always enjoyed good health. Of late, however, she has become increasingly tired. She feels 'run down', has difficulty concentrating, and feels somewhat low in mood. Of course, her long hours at work are the most obvious explanation for her fatigue, but further questioning proved very rewarding. It turns out that she feels particularly tired after eating meals, especially if these consisted of cake or biscuits, sugar-laden foods. She also noticed that these foods sometimes make her feel dizzy shortly after ingestion. Furthermore, because she only gets six hours' sleep a night, she drinks seven mugs of coffee and ten mugs of tea to keep herself awake during the day. That's a total of 3 grams of alkaloid daily! She also smokes ten cigarettes each day, usually with her cups of caffeine! To complicate matters, she became a vegetarian three years ago, and was probably not in a good nutritional state.

Lara demonstrates a few salient features. She was sleep deprived, stressed, she was drinking vast quantities of caffeine, smoked cigarettes, and had symptoms of hypoglycaemia. She was, incidentally, conscientious but not thin or 'hyperkinetic', tenacious but not compulsive, concerned about her fatigue but not intense.

It is interesting to note her reactions to carbohydrate foods.

They made her feel tired and dizzy, well-known symptoms of the postprandial syndrome. Of course, the amount of caffeine, nicotine and adrenaline in her system would only aggravate this problem, as well as causing symptoms in their own right. Lara was advised to (i) sleep regular hours, (ii) reduce caffeine intake, (iii) avoid cigarettes as much as possible, (iv) eat six small, nutritionally balanced meals per day, and (v) avoid excessive sugars. She quickly regained the full strength of her body and mind.

18 *The Truth about Candida*

Candida has received a great deal of attention in recent years, and has earned a rather dubious reputation in the public mind. It is said to be the cause of an untold number of human ills. All manner of symptoms have been attributed to it, from temper outbursts to impotence. In fact, if you read through the non-medical books on the subject, you will find at least fifty different symptoms blamed on candida. The medical community, on the other hand, is not so concerned. It recognises that candida can cause oral, skin and genital infections, of course, but these respond very rapidly to treatment. It further recognises that patients with compromised immune systems are prone to more serious and widespread candida infection. Apart from these clearly understood infections, doctors generally consider candida to be an innocent bystander. Let's take a closer look at this contentious issue.

What is candida?

Candida is a family of yeast. In fact, it is a rather large family consisting of at least 200 different species, brothers and sisters so to speak. The most important of these, from a human point of view, is *Candida albicans*. This yeast inhabits the mouth, gastrointestinal tract, vagina and skin of healthy humans. There is nothing unusual about this, for many micro-organisms inhabit our bodies in this way. The relationship we have with these, our resident microbes, is a symbiotic one: they scratch our back; and we scratch theirs. We provide them with a place to live and nutrients to live on; and they, in return, provide us with several important services, including (a) assistance with digestion, (b) provision of some vitamins, and (c) some degree of protection from more harmful microbes. Our resident microbial colonies compete with each other for space and food. This is healthy competition. It ensures that an ecological balance is struck between bedfellows, and in the context of this chapter, it ensures that the candida yeasts are held in check. The immune system, meanwhile, keeps a watchful, balancing eye on all this ecological pushing and shoving. In summary, then, we all have candida. And, in health, it is an innocent bystander. Having thus rescued its reputation, it must be said that candida can cause several problems: we can be allergic to it, we can be infected by it, and we can have too much of it. The latter condition is of particular relevance to fatigue.

Candida allergy

Some people are allergic to candida. There is no doubt about this. Urticaria, rhinitis, and asthma are sometimes triggered by this allergen. The medical literature also contains indisputable descriptions of candida allergy in the bowel and genitalia. These are less well-known entities, but very real none the less.

Candida allergy in the bowel	causes 'mucous colitis', a condition characterised by slimy and sometimes profuse diarrhoea.
Candida allergy in the vagina	causes vaginitis, an inflammation which looks like infection. The symptoms include pain, itch and redness.
Candida allergy on the penis	causes inflammation. The symptoms are itch, pain and swelling.

Note: In all these cases, a skin prick test to candida will be positive, and the patient will enjoy dramatic symptomatic relief from anti-candida treatment.

Candida infections

Candida albicans can cause infection under certain circumstances. It changes from a normal inhabitant to an infective agent when the ecological status quo is lost. The most obvious example of this is vaginal (or oral) thrush that so frequently follows a course of antibiotics. The antibiotic kills the germ it was intended to kill, but it also kills off many innocent bacteria. Candida, on the other hand, being resistant to ordinary antibiotics, grows away happily in their presence. It has no competition from other bacteria, so it just keeps on growing. Before long it causes symptoms of infection. In this sense, candida can truly be called an opportunistic agent: it has no ability of its own to invade, and will only infect if given the opportunity to do so. There are three types of opportunistic infection caused by candida. These are described as superficial, deep and systemic. Deep and systemic (blood-borne) invasions only ever occur in patients who are immuno-compromised, such as patients with AIDS, or those seriously ill with some other disease. Superficial infections, by contrast, are very common. As the name suggests, the invasion is limited to superficial layers of the surface being infected. Commonly affected sites include the skin, mouth and vagina; less commonly affected are the linings of the throat, oesophagus, stomach and bowel.

CANDIDA ON THE SKIN

Candida infections of the skin may occur at any age, but there are two age groups that are particularly prone. Children under 3 years of age, for example, easily develop candida infections in the nappy area, giving them anything from a mild irritation to a rather nasty dermatitis. The second group at risk are adolescents who take antibiotics for recurrent urinary or throat infections, or acne. The principal symptom of candida infection of the skin is an itchy rash which may, at its worst, become excoriated and sore. The infection most frequently affects the skin folds (where it's warm and moist), such as the armpits, the groin and the spaces between toes or fingers. The nails too may be affected.

CANDIDA IN THE MOUTH

Oral infections occur in all age groups, but again some groups are more at risk than others. Seven per cent of infants, for example, get oral candida (thrush). They are prone to infection because their immune systems are immature, and they have not had enough time to establish an ecological balance with other friendly microbes. The elderly are also commonly affected, possibly because of the ageing process itself, and in some cases because of ill-fitting dentures. Finally, diabetic patients, whose sugar levels are too high, and patients who inhale steroids for their asthma, are more likely to develop infection. The main symptom of oral thrush is pain, especially when eating salty or spicy foods. Other symptoms include (a) sores at the corners of the mouth, (b) inflamed mucous membranes inside the mouth, (c) white creamy plaques on the tongue and on the inner aspect of the lips, cheeks and palate, and (d) mouth ulcers.

CANDIDA IN THE VAGINA

Candida infections in the vagina are extremely common, with 75 per cent of women experiencing at least one bout during their child-bearing years. Half of these can expect a second infection at a later date. The universal symptom of vaginal candida is itch. This may or may not be accompanied by a vaginal discharge which, if present, is said to be white and creamy (a bit like cottage cheese), but it may also assume a watery appearance. Other symptoms include vaginal soreness, painful intercourse and bladder pain when passing water. The latter is frequently mistaken for cystitis (a bladder infection), but this symptom arises from an irritation of the bladder neck, rather than from a bladder infection *per se*. Treatment is usually very successful. Having said that, 5 per cent of adult females are plagued by recurrent or chronic infection. Some of these may be infected with a candida species other than albicans, such as *Candida tropicalis*, for example. The latter is rare but becoming more common, and it's more resistant to treatment. However, and bearing in mind the fact that candida is an opportunistic fellow, it is more likely that patients with a recurrent infection are struggling with their internal ecological balance. Factors which alter the balance and predispose to vaginal infection include:

174

- Pregnancy.
- Oral contraceptives, especially those with high doses of oestrogen.
- Antibiotics, especially the broad-spectrum (blunderbuss) ones.
- Steroids.
- Allergy in the vagina, to perfumed toilet paper, for example.
- Certain diseases, such as *Diabetes mellitus*.

Other factors which may be important include:

- Tight clothing, especially nylons which prevent adequate ventilation.
- Eating lots of sugary foods.
- Vaginal douches.
- Swimming in chlorinated pools.
- Intra-uterine contraceptive devices (IUCDs).
- Frequency of sexual intercourse.
- Reinfection from an untreated sexual partner.
- Reinfection from a reservoir of candida in the bowel (see below).

Bacterial and other vaginal infections are twice as common as vaginal thrush. The only way to make sure that you are, in fact, dealing with thrush, and not some other infective agent, is by having a vaginal swab test. Also, the symptoms of *allergic* vaginal inflammation are very similar to the symptoms of *infective* inflammation. For this reason allergy is often overlooked and mistaken for infection. The transient relief which candida-allergic women enjoy from anti-candida treatments only adds to the confusion. They feel they must have an infection because their symptoms clear up with treatment. The real reason for their relief, however, is the reduction of vaginal candida as an *allergen* rather than as an *infective agent*. The clue is the disparity between the symptoms and the presence of yeast. Allergic symptoms may be severe in the absence of a significant vaginal discharge, and in the presence of only a small amount of candida. Patients with recurrent vaginal infections should have a skin prick test to exclude candida allergy. They should also read the rest of this chapter!

175

CANDIDA IN THE BOWEL

We have already established that candida is a normal inhabitant of the bowel, and that its numbers are kept in check by other microbes with which it must compete. Once again, there are several factors which may upset this balance and predispose to candida overgrowth. These are:

- being very young or very old
- recurrent pregnancies
- the oral contraceptive pill
- taking antibiotics
- eating a diet of sugary foods
- vitamin deficiency
- having a stomach lacking in acid (hypochlorhydria)
- taking remedies for indigestion or stomach ulcers (antacids)
- taking steroids
- stress.

Candida infections in the bowel, as elsewhere, may take on superficial or deep forms, and I stress again that the latter only ever occur in the seriously ill. The symptoms of infection include diarrhoea, flatulence, abdominal pain, rectal bleeding and an itchy bum. No other symptoms occur — except in moribund, and usually hospitalised, patients whose immune defences have collapsed entirely. However, we need to understand that candida overgrowth is not synonymous with candida infection. This is important. They are two different conditions: infection implies some attempt by the organism to invade tissue; whereas overgrowth refers simply to a population explosion without invading qualities. We are particularly interested in this phenomenon because it gives rise, potentially, to two problems. The first was alluded to above, namely, that increased numbers of candida constitute a rich reservoir for recurrent vaginal infections. Note the sequence of events here. The distance between rectum and vagina is short and easily breached by the imaginative yeast. To treat the vagina repeatedly whilst ignoring the intestinal reservoir is to fight a losing battle, for no sooner has the vagina been cleared than it becomes infected again through this route. Please also note that hygiene has little or nothing to do with it! Recurrent infections are not a sign of 'dirtiness'; they occur just as frequently in meticulously clean individuals. The one sanitary precaution which females should adopt in this regard is to wipe the bottom from front to back after a bowel movement.

The second major problem of candida overgrowth is the gut fermentation syndrome. This condition may affect both men and women, and it may occur with or without genital infections. As you will see, gut fermentation may be caused by any number of different microbes. Candida, although commonly implicated, is just one candidate. There are many other yeasts and bacteria that can drive the fermenting process.

Gut fermentation syndrome: intestinal dysbiosis

We have described symbiosis as a relationship of mutual benefit between one organism and another, or between several organisms and a host. In this context, we are talking of the friendly relationship that exists between our bodies and the myriad microbes which live inside us. Indeed, there are an estimated 100,000 million microbes in each gram of faeces! In health, these microscopic residents are maintained in a state of balance. If this equilibrium is lost, for whatever reason, one micro-organism will grow at the expense of others. The diplomatic relationship between host and organism is now less harmonious than before. We refer to this as a state of dysbiosis. Furthermore, if the expanding microbe just so happens to be capable of fermentation, it may give rise to symptoms. Several bacteria and yeasts fall into this category. They live by fermenting the sugars in our diet, that is, they set to work on 'eating' the sugars, and they produce alcohol as a by-product. Some fermentation takes place inside all of us, and there are usually no problems with this. But if the fermenting population becomes unacceptably large, the fermentation process — the feeding frenzy, as it were — also increases dramatically. Now we have a situation where alcohol and other products of fermentation, such as gas and toxins, are released into the bowel. Alcohol and toxins are then absorbed into the bloodstream from whence they cause a lot of misery. In extreme (and very rare) cases, patients have been known to intoxicate themselves by eating carbohydrate foods, i.e. they can get drunk on sugars!

The symptoms of gut fermentation include:

- Abdominal pain
- Altered stool frequency
- Altered stool form
- Altered stool passage
- Passing mucus from the back passage
- Bloating of the abdomen
- Itchy bottom
- Flatulence
- Indigestion.

As you may know, these symptoms overlap greatly with those of irritable bowel syndrome. This has to do with the direct effect of microbial overgrowth and fermentation on bowel function. These are 'local' symptoms. The absorption of alcohol and other toxins into the blood gives rise to 'distant' symptoms, namely

- fatigue
- headache
- muscle pain
- joint pain.

Furthermore, some patients attribute their depression, disturbed sleep and impaired concentration to excessive fermentation. Whilst I fully accept that these symptoms are often part of the overall picture, it is difficult to separate them from the reactive effects of feeling ill for so long. But the notion that fermentation causes 'brain symptoms' is not as daft as it may first appear. Acetaldehyde, for example, is a by-product of fermentation and is known to affect a specific (dopamine) receptor in brain cells. In any case, these troublesome symptoms clear up once the fermentation is treated.

You will also appreciate that many of these symptoms may be caused by food intolerance, or indeed any number of other conditions. In days gone by we had no option but to put patients on a lengthy diet if we suspected they had fermentation, and patients had to wait some considerable time before they knew whether they would benefit from treatment. Our task is now greatly facilitated by the recent development of a blood test.

A blood test for gut fermentation

Microbes produce alcohol when they ferment sugars. Specifically, yeasts produce ethanol,[1] and bacteria produce butanol and propanol. We can measure these different alcohols in the blood. If the levels are raised, we can deduce that excessive fermentation is taking place; and, depending on the type of alcohol produced, we can say whether the fermentation is of yeast or bacterial origin. However, we cannot specify which yeast or bacterium is responsible for the fermentation. But that's OK — we don't need to know. There is one treatment for yeast fermentation, whatever the yeast, and another for bacterial fermentation, whatever the bacteria. Here are a few examples.

Case histories

Pauline was a very busy person with a very important job. She was responsible for the day-to-day management of a large company. Over the past five years she had suffered from recurrent vaginal infections. Swab tests confirmed that she was infected with candida. She had become quite fed up with the vaginal itch and pain. Symptoms persisted in spite of frequent prescriptions from her doctor. Her husband was also treated on a number of occasions 'just in case'. Pauline suddenly became very unwell about six months before she presented to the clinic. She was exhausted. She also developed pains in her muscles and joints. Her back, shoulders and arms were affected in this way. At one stage she was so ill that she slept sixteen hours a day for the best part of three weeks. In addition, she complained of bouts of diarrhoea, abdominal pain, an itchy bottom and indigestion. She lost a stone in weight. Throughout this time her vaginal infections continued unabated. In fact, she now had chronic vaginal symptoms. A blood test revealed that Pauline was suffering from the effects of yeast overgrowth in the bowel. She was put on a diet, and she was prescribed antifungal medication to take by mouth. One month later, and already feeling considerably better in herself, she was given antifungal treatment for the vaginal infections. Over the following weeks and months she expanded her diet bit by bit.

1. You may not know it, but you are probably familiar with this alcohol already — it's the intoxicating part of your favourite drink!

At the time of writing she remains well, and she has had only one bout of vaginal thrush in the past eight months.

Fred too was a busy person, and had a very demanding job. Over the previous three or four years he had complained of increasing fatigue. He also complained of abdominal symptoms, such as bloating and diarrhoea. He thought that certain foods were making him ill. In particular, he discovered that all forms of sugar affected him. The problem for Fred, however, was his craving for the very foods that 'wiped him out'. He underwent a low allergy diet for ten days and, although he felt somewhat better, he still had quite a few symptoms left. It was clear that his problem was not food intolerance. A blood test for fermentation was then arranged, which came back positive. In fact, the alcohol level in his fasting blood was forty times higher than it should have been! He was started on a regime of diet and antifungal medication. Fred simply could not believe the improvement in his health once he controlled his fermentation. It took a little longer in his case, because the levels were so high. Pauline and Fred had yeast fermentation. Notice I didn't say they had candida! Their fermentation may have been caused by candida, but it may just as easily have been caused by other yeasts in the gut.

Andrea was different. She suffered from recurrent urinary infections, and had taken twenty courses of antibiotic in as many months! During this time she developed many other symptoms, including fatigue, headaches, fitful sleep, impaired memory and concentration, muscle pains and joint pains. Interestingly, she had little by way of abdominal symptoms. However, in view of her inordinate consumption of antibiotics and the timing of her symptoms, we performed a gut fermentation test. This revealed the presence of bacterial fermentation. Her butanol levels were about ten times higher than they should have been. She was given antibacterial medication (but not an antibiotic!) together with the gut fermentation diet.

Within a month she felt better, and within three months she was back to her old self. When she started to expand her diet again, she reacted to wheat and a few other foods. Thus Andrea had a combination of gut fermentation and food intolerance.

This is quite a common occurrence. And, as you will see in Chapter 20, gut fermentation is also associated with chemical sensitivity.

The treatment of gut fermentation syndrome

The aim of treatment is to restore balance among micro-organisms in the gut. To this end, we must reduce the overgrown population to normal numbers. We do not need to eradicate them completely; nor do we want to. We respect that, in the right numbers, they provide us with many benefits. Besides, we couldn't get rid of them all; they're too versatile for that! A simple culling will suffice. To do this we employ four tactics:

1. We restrict our intake of sugars, thus depriving the microbe of its favourite food (and ours).
2. We use medication to further reduce the microbial population.
3. We replace the fermenting microbe with friendly bacteria.
4. We use nutritional supplements to help our immune systems.

The only difference between the treatment of yeast and bacterial fermentation is in the use of medication. The principles of diet, microbial replacement and nutritional supplement are the same.

THE GUT FERMENTATION DIET (STAGE 1)

You will find variations on this theme in various books, some of them stricter than others. Mine is fairly relaxed by comparison. The diet applies to both yeast and bacterial fermentation. For the first month you should eat *only* the following (preferably fresh) foods:

- Meat: all sorts: lamb, pork, beef, venison, rabbit etc.
- Poultry: all sorts: chicken, turkey, pheasant, duck, quail etc.
- Fish: all sorts: including shellfish, but must be fresh, not in batter.
- Vegetables: all sorts (except sweetcorn and peas which are high in sugar). Eat plenty of greens and garlic (which has known antifungal properties). Potato and rice are good carbohydrate foods and should be eaten in moderation, say,

two helpings per day. You can also use rice cakes.

- Fruit: two normal portions of your choice per day.
- Beans & pulses: all sorts, but in moderation (kidney beans, lentils, sunflower seeds etc.).
- Cheese: Edam and Gouda cheese are allowed, as is goat's cheese.
- Live yoghurt: and plenty of it (see below).
- Eggs and butter.
- Use olive oil for cooking purposes.
- Drink only bottled (or filtered) spring water, herbal teas and calcium-fortified soy milk.
- Take medication, nutritional supplements and friendly bacteria as prescribed, and continue on these throughout the entire process (see below).
- Obviously, if you know you are allergic to any of the above, stay away from them.

THE GUT FERMENTATION DIET (STAGE 2)

You should have noticed some improvement in the symptoms by the end of the first month. You can now expand your diet. However, some of the improvement may have been due to the fact that you stopped eating food(s) to which you are intolerant. It would be wise then to introduce these foods one by one and observe your reaction to them as you do so (see the low allergy diet in Chapter 15 for more details on this). Continue to eat all the stage 1 foods throughout this time and test each new food as follows:

THE GUT FERMENTATION DIET (STAGE 3)

By now you should be well and truly on the road to recovery. If you are, try out the following over the coming month: all kinds of cheese (including mouldy ones), tea and coffee, all sorts of nuts, and alcohol. Later, you may also venture towards cake, biscuits, chocolate, ice cream, rich sauces etc.

Please accept two pieces of advice before we leave the subject of diet. Firstly, if you have not enjoyed obvious and lasting benefit within two months of this regime, then *something is wrong!* The diagnosis should be reconsidered in such cases. Please resist the urge to stay on this or any other diet, unless it has been advised by

The gut fermentation diet (stage 2)	
Day 1	Cow's milk: drink one glass at each meal for one day.
Days 2, 3 and 4	Wheat in the form of (i) wholemeal pasta (ii) pure shredded wheat (iii) wholemeal bread. Some form of wheat must be eaten at each meal for the three full days. The bread should ideally be home made, using wholemeal flour — no white flour added. Use bread soda and add an egg if you like. You may also use buttermilk, if milk is safe.
Day 5	Peanuts in the form of (i) peanut butter (with no added sugar) (i) raw monkey nuts (i) salted peanuts. Stay away from dry roasted nuts. Eat some form of peanut at each meal for one day.
Days 6 and 7	Corn in the form of: (i) corn on the cob (i) home-made popcorn (i) cornflour, to make a sauce. Eat some form of corn at each meal for two full days.
Days 8 and 9	Oats in the form of (i) porridge (i) oatcakes. Eat some form of oats at each meal for two full days.
Days 10 and 11	Rye in the form of (i) ryvita crispbread (i) pure rye bread. Eat some rye at each meal for two full days.

your doctor/dietician. Secondly, watch out for a return of the symptoms as you reintroduce sugary foods. These symptoms are likely to creep up on you gradually as the fermentation builds up. Once again, please get expert help if you find this happening. I believe that the vast majority of patients with fermentation can end up with a normal or nearly normal diet. In other words, gut fermentation is a treatable disorder with a high rate of cure. You would, of course, be well advised to eat a healthy diet for the rest of your days. This will mean some degree of moderation in your consumption of sugars, but it will also allow the occasional splurge!

Drug treatment for gut fermentation

The choice of drug is dictated by the organism we are dealing with. Yeast can be tackled head on with antifungal drugs, whereas we must take a more subtle approach with bacterial overgrowth.

YEAST FERMENTATION

The most effective medicine for the treatment of yeast fermentation is nystatin, a powerful antifungal drug. This is taken, ideally, in the form of a powder. All other preparations of nystatin are sugar laden. Fortunately, nystatin is also a very safe drug and can be taken in large doses without ill effects. Its safety and efficacy stem from the fact that its absorption into the body is negligible. This serves our purpose well. We want it to stay in the gut.

Some patients complain that it makes them feel ill, and there is no doubt that a minority of these are genuinely intolerant to the drug itself. But most of the symptoms attributed to nystatin actually come from the dying yeast colonies. Yeast cells burst when they die, and their contents spill out into the gut. Some of these substances are toxic to us, and they give rise to flu-like symptoms, such as headache, fatigue, and aches and pains in the muscles. These die-off reactions, as they're called, can be minimised by starting with very small doses of nystatin, with gradual increases until therapeutic (effective) levels are reached. Starting the diet a week before the nystatin will also help, for this will (slightly) reduce yeast populations in itself. Nystatin is a prescription-only medicine, so discuss its use with your doctor. I recommend the following dosage schedule:

Dosing schedule for dry nystatin powder

Start with:
: 1/8 level teaspoon per day for three days — literally the tip of a level teaspoon.

Then double to:
: 1/4 level tsp per day for three days.

Then double to:
: 1/2 level tsp per day for seven days.

Then double to:
: 1 level tsp per day. I usually advise patients to stay on this dose for a total of three months, and only rarely have to give larger doses.

Note: The powder does not taste nice! Mix your daily dose into live yoghurt, store it in the fridge and dip into it several times a day. Die-off reactions may occur when you start nystatin, and at any dose increase thereafter. If you get die-off symptoms, grin and bear them, as they will pass. If they're too severe, go back to the previous dose and try to increase the dose again in another week.

A WORD ABOUT OTHER ANTIFUNGALS

Nystatin is the most suitable medication for yeast fermentation, but some patients (a minority) are intolerant to it. They get symptoms even when they observe the dosing precautions just described. These require an alternative antifungal. All such treatments are prescription-only medicines. They are absorbed into the bloodstream and are therefore less effective than nystatin in the treatment of fermentation. They are very effective for the treatment of infection, however. The use of these drugs should be discussed with your doctor. Some individuals and health food shops sell stuff which is supposedly antifungal. The truth is, they *limit* the ability of yeast to grow, but they don't kill them off. If you have a significant overgrowth, you will need a 'killer', not a 'limiter'. Once the overgrowth is controlled, then by all means use these yeast-limiting agents to prevent a recurrence.

BACTERIAL FERMENTATION

Bacterial overgrowth cannot be tackled head-on with antibiotics. That would only make matters worse! There is one exception to this rule — young childrem with severe upper gastrointestinal overgrowth respond well to antibiotics. For the rest of us, we rely on an old drug, bismuth. This medicine was popular in times past for the treatment of gastritis and ulcers, and is still used today. It is thought to work by lining the stomach with a protective coat. When bismuth lines the stomach and intestine, it acts rather like grease on a pole: it's very hard for bacteria to cling on to the bowel wall. They lose their grip, slip off, and get expelled from the body in the faeces. We use Denoltab, a tablet containing bismuth. It should not be taken for longer than three months at a time because it's absorbed into the bloodstream. Two tablets taken half an hour before breakfast and evening meals is the recommended dose. (It turns the stool black!)

FRIENDLY BACTERIA TO RESTORE THE BALANCE

Once we kill off the fermenting organism, we must fill the empty space with friendly bacteria. This will ensure that the fermenting organism is held in check. The best way to achieve this is to flood the gut with friendly bacteria, such as those we find in live yoghurt. They go by some wonderful names, such as *bulgaricus*, *lactobacillus* and *bifidus*. Choose a brand that guarantees live bacteria, and eat one good-sized pot of it every day. Some brands boast two or more cultures of bacteria. These are the best, for they provide a variety which can only help the ecological balance of the gut.

You should verify that your chosen yoghurt is truly alive by the following simple test. Place a desertspoon of milk on top of a newly opened pot of yoghurt, put the top back on, and place it in a warm oven. Come back in five hours and observe that the milk has disappeared. If it hasn't, the live culture is in fact dead! Supplements of friendly bacteria are also available. One of the most popular of these is acidophilus. However, beware of the claims — many of the acidophilus are dead by the time they reach your local supplier!

Nutritional supplements to help our immune systems

Yeasts grow more vehemently in the absence of certain vitamins. They also grow more readily in the absence of an effective immune system. The B vitamins are important in this regard, so take a supplement of B complex throughout the diet. Other nutrients may also help, but these should be determined on an individual basis.

Candida hypersensitivity syndrome

I come back now to my opening paragraph, in which I pointed out that all manner of ills have been blamed on candida. Some practitioners refer to this plethora of symptoms as the candida hypersensitivity syndrome, or candida, for short. Their list is far more extensive than the symptoms I have described above, and there are two sources of confusion here. The first is the commercial interest of unqualified practitioners who forcibly tell clients that their unexplained symptoms are due to candida — and then sell them the wherewithal to treat it! The second is this: the popular treatment for candida involves killing several birds with one stone. Potentially allergic foods (such as wheat and yeast) are avoided; pharmacologically active foods (such as caffeine and alcohol) are avoided; potentially 'tiring' foods (sugars) are avoided; and nutritional supplements are taken in large doses. These measures, *in and of themselves*, would improve the health of many.

Thus, the candida regime could help the food intolerant, the caffeine addicted, the postprandial, the nutritionally deficient and the gut-fermenting. As you can see, the fact that you improve on a candida regime does not necessarily prove that your symptoms were caused by candida. But one can readily understand this source of confusion.

You will notice that all the symptoms attributed to candida in this chapter can be verified by clinical and laboratory tests, and by their speedy response to appropriate treatment. I would encourage anyone with persistent symptoms to seek expert help and, if need be, to think again about the diagnosis of candida. When all is said and done, most patients should end up with a clear understanding of the true nature of their symptoms. This will afford them the best possible chance of obtaining relief.

Parasites, Bacteria

19 and Viruses

By definition, a parasite is an organism that lives in (or on) an unwilling host, and derives its food and shelter from it. Although yeasts, bacteria and viruses are, strictly speaking, parasites, medical tradition reserves everyday usage of the term for much larger organisms known as protozoa and helminths. Protozoa are, in spite of their greater size, not visible to the naked eye, whereas helminths, being much larger again, are. Helminths are colloquially known as 'worms'. They are often recognised as such on the stools of infected persons.

On a global scale parasites are the single most common cause of fatigue and debility. Malaria, for example, is a protozoan infection (*plasmodium spp*) which affects in the region of a million new people each year. Similarly, bilharzia is a disease caused by helminths of the *schistosoma spp*. There are well in excess of 100 million infected people worldwide. These are of course tropical diseases, and they are only seen in Western society among travellers returning from affected countries. It is now easier than ever to travel around the world, and many do so for both business and pleasure purposes. If your fatigue started after a trip abroad, you should consider the possibility that you have picked up an unwelcome parasitic guest, even if you did not suffer an acute illness during your stay abroad.

It is, however, quite possible, and indeed common, to pick up parasites without ever leaving home! Some parasites are cosmopolitan — they have managed to infiltrate and establish a presence in every country in the world. Some of these are well known for their propensity to cause tummy upsets, but some of them have also been implicated in chronic fatigue. Indeed, some patients have been mistakenly diagnosed as suffering from chronic fatigue syndrome, only to discover later that their real problem was parasites. Parasites go by some beautiful names: *Giardia lamblia*, *Blastocystis hominis*, *Entamoeba coli*, *Endolimax nana* and *Dientamoeba fragilis*, to name but a few. The discerning reader will recognise that I have included parasites which have been traditionally thought of as being normal commensals, i.e. harmless. They are included here because of mounting evidence that they do indeed cause disease. They are not the innocent bystanders we once thought they were!

Intestinal parasites

SILENT CARRIAGE

Parasites are capable of setting up home in a bowel without ever causing symptoms. Indeed, they may persist for years on end without causing trouble to their host. Having established themselves in residence, they produce offspring to their hearts' content; these are excreted in the faeces and passed on to the next unsuspecting host through contaminated food and water. The whole life cycle may proceed without causing symptoms. This is called the 'silent carrier' state. Because of this well-recognised phenomenon of asymptomatic carriage, it was initially thought that many of these organisms were not pathogenic to man. However, this tenet has been severely challenged in the recent past.

ACUTE INFECTION

Parasites may cause acute abdominal symptoms upon their first attempt to invade a bowel. The body reacts by producing a profuse diarrhoea (in the hope of flushing out the parasite). This may be accompanied by fever, flu-like pains and other symptoms. The immune system will try its best to eradicate the parasite, but may not succeed. If it fails, the parasite becomes firmly established and the symptoms of chronic infection may ensue.

CHRONIC INFECTION

As you would expect, the commonest symptoms of chronic intestinal parasite infection are gastrointestinal: diarrhoea (or alternating diarrhoea and constipation), bloating of the abdomen, hunger pangs, chronic indigestion, abdominal pain (which may be severe enough to mimic an ulcer), flatulence and an itchy anus. The stools become watery or semi-solid, greasy, bulky and foul smelling. They may be pale in colour and float on the water in the toilet bowl (because of the undigested fats), and they may be difficult to flush. However, it is possible for a parasite to cause a great deal of ill health *without* causing tell-tale abdominal symptoms. This diagnosis must therefore be borne in mind when seeking relief from chronic fatigue.

Apart from these local symptoms, there may also be profound lassitude, headache, muscle pain and weakness, sore throats, swollen glands, joint pains, depression and recurrent low-grade fevers. In some cases there is a gradual loss of appetite and malabsorption of nutrients. These will lead to significant nutritional deficiencies, and the symptoms of malnutrition will then complicate the picture.

ALLERGY AND OTHER EFFECTS ON THE IMMUNE SYSTEM

The successful parasite will burrow its way into the lining of the bowel wall and remain there in comfort for years. The host, however, will not be so comfortable! On the one hand his immune system is suppressed by the parasite, and on the other he may become allergic to it. This gives rise to allergic reactions such as urticaria, as well as local reactions in the bowel wall. Furthermore, the intestinal micro-flora are disturbed by its presence, and yeast such as candida is allowed to proliferate. Now we have a dual infection. Add to this the subsequent development of food allergies or intolerance, which are commonly seen with both candida and parasite infections, and we end up with a very ill patient indeed. Such patients may suffer the cumulative effects of the local and systemic symptoms of parasitic and yeast infection, together with the symptoms of food allergy, nutritional deficiency and chemical sensitivity.

Making a diagnosis

Parasitic infection should be considered a possibility in all patients who have unresolved intestinal symptoms and/or chronic fatigue.

Unfortunately, and in spite of an increasing interest in parasites, it still happens that such patients have to undergo extensive investigation before the diagnosis is even considered. They should have a test to confirm or exclude the presence of parasites in the bowel. Admittedly, merely identifying a parasite does not prove that it is responsible for the fatigue; but because we know it can be, we should make every effort to eradicate it.

The traditional diagnostic approach has been to examine stool samples under a microscope for eggs, but this has proved to be a woefully inadequate test. Even rampant infections may not show up with this method. One documented case, in which the small intestine was known to be absolutely riddled with parasites, had over thirty consecutive negative stool samples! Part of the reason for such failure may be that the older staining techniques did not detect the organisms (staining involves washing the sample with various dyes in the hope that these would be absorbed into the parasite, thus enabling the investigator to identify it by virtue of its colour). But it is equally possible that there were no parasites to be seen in the stool itself. By the time they got to the large bowel, they may have burrowed their way into the wall. Negative stool samples *do not* provide sufficient evidence to exclude infection. The definitive investigation for parasitic infection is to conduct a biopsy of the small intestine in the laboratory, but biopsies of this sort are invasive, that is, they constitute a surgical procedure. More recently, vigorous swabs taken from the rectal wall are being examined with a more sensitive stain. The swab is taken painlessly through an anoscope, an instrument used for the visualisation of the anal canal and lower rectum. This procedure is not nearly as invasive as a biopsy, and so far it shows promising results.

Treatments for intestinal parasites

Intestinal parasites must be treated actively with antiparasitic medication. The usual first choice of drug is metronidazole. This should be taken over a ten day period. It may make you feel nauseated, and it sometimes leaves a metallic taste in your mouth during treatment. There are herbal alternatives such as *Artemisia annua* extract, which is given in a dose of 1,000 mg three times a day for up to three months, and grapefruit seed extract, which is given in a dose of 150–300 mg three times a day for up to three months. Some parasites are particularly resistant to treatment. If one of the above-mentioned therapies fails to control the infection, it should be treated with two or more medicines simultaneously, and for a prolonged period. Attention must also be paid to concurrent candida overgrowth and nutritional deficiencies.

Case history

Amy was 50 years old by the time I saw her. She had been unwell for about four years. Her symptoms started after an acute flu-like illness which was characterised by high fever, aches and pains all over, nausea and prostration. She was admitted to hospital for investigation and treatment, but no cause was ever found for her illness, and she had remained unwell ever since. Her main symptoms, as presented to me, were overwhelming fatigue, nausea, bloating of the abdomen, pruritus ani, and diarrhoea productive of foul-smelling, pale, semi-solid stools that floated on the water and were difficult to flush. In addition, she had joint pains, headaches, a disturbed sleep pattern, urticaria, and a peculiar burning sensation in her feet.

A rectal swab revealed that she was heavily infected with *Blastocystis hominis*. She was given a course of metronidazole which made no difference to herself, or to her rectal parasite population. She was then treated with grapefruit seed extract over a thirty day period. This did seem to help her symptoms somwhat, but she was still fatigued and suffered ongoing bowel symptoms. A third swab performed at this point showed that there was still a significant parasitic presence, so she was prescribed a combination of artemisia, grapefruit seed extract, together with a third medicine (diloxanide furoate). Over the ninety days of treatment, she made steady progress toward a full and energetic life, free of symptoms.

Some other germs of importance to the fatigued

Toxoplasmosis

Toxoplasmosis is a disease caused by the small parasite *Toxoplasma gondii*. The manifestations of toxoplasma infection are varied and range from devastating life-threatening disease to having no symptoms at all. Indeed, large portions of the population have been infected with toxoplasma at some stage in the past — without ever realising it. If they did have symptoms, they were so mild as to escape notice, or they were mistaken for a mild viral infection. What is of interest to us, in the context of fatigue, is that toxoplasma may cause a disease very similar to glandular fever, called 'acquired toxoplasmosis'. This is characterised by fatigue, swollen glands, muscle pain and low-grade fevers. Diagnosis is rather complex and depends on the expert interpretation of blood tests.

This parasite has a particular liking for domestic cats! It seems that this is the only animal in which it can multiply. Infections are acquired from contact with cat faeces, or by the ingestion of raw or undercooked, infected meat. *Toxocara* is a similar parasite carried by dogs.

Brucellosis

This is a disease caused by the *Brucella* bacteria. It is acquired from contact with infected animals, or by ingestion of infected dairy products such as butter and milk. It is an occupational hazard for farmers, meat-packers and veterinarians. It may start abruptly or very gradually. The acute presentation is characterised by fever, thumping headaches, muscular pains, malaise and (occasionally) diarrhoea. Most uncomplicated cases settle within a matter of weeks without serious consequences. However, there is a chronic form of the disease characterised by fatigue, recurrent fevers, headaches, joint pains, back pain, constipation, abdominal pain, irritable and/or depressed mood, insomnia and emotional lability. As you will see, many of these symptoms also occur in chronic fatigue syndrome (CFS). The importance of the distinction is that brucellosis may respond to antibiotic therapy, whereas CFS does not.

Q fever

Q fever is caused by a bug from the Rickettsial family called *Coxsiella burnetti*. The principal sources are domestic and farm animals. The disease is acquired by inhalation of microscopic droplets of infected material in the air near infected animals (which may have no symptoms of illness themselves). It may also be contracted through tick bites. The clinical symptoms include fever, severe headache, extreme fatigue, muscle pain and chest pain with a dry cough. Most cases recover without problems after a few weeks, but a few go on to develop chronic fatigue. In rare cases the heart is affected, but in the vast majority there are no signs of physical disease. There is a growing consensus among doctors of the existence of a genuine chronic fatigue state following some cases of Q fever.

Tuberculosis

Tuberculosis (TB) is a chronic infection caused by mycobacteria. Infection is acquired most commonly by the inhalation of infected cough droplets that may remain suspended in the air for long periods. For this reason, one silent carrier can infect an entire environment such as a school or workplace, with the risk of infection persisting even after they have been removed. Many people exposed to TB don't know they have it — the infection remains dormant, sometimes for years. A precarious stand-off occurs between body and bug. The body manages to keep the infection isolated in small pockets called foci, but the bug struggles to multiply even within these foci. Nutrition, general health and psychosocial factors are important in this battle. Any extra burden, such as concurrent illness, immuno-suppressant drugs, nutritional deficiency, or even stress, could tip the balance in favour of the infection. Symptoms will occur as soon as the infection has gained the upper hand. Our interest lies in the fact that the early symptoms are entirely non-specific. Fatigue features prominently in this context, although loss of appetite, night sweats and weight loss may also occur. Treatment with antibiotics has greatly improved the outlook for patients with TB.

Lyme disease

So called because of clusters of a mysterious illness that affected several communities in eastern Connecticut, USA. It was several years before a clever chap by the name of Burgdorfer discovered the bug responsible for the disease. It turned out to be a spirochete, christened *Borellia burgdorferi*. The bug is transmitted by ticks that have previously fed on infected animals, such as deer. Lyme disease occurs in three distinct phases. Stage 1 is a characteristic skin rash called *Erythema chronicum migrans* (ECM). This develops at the site of the tick bite, and looks like a raised, red (*erythema*) circle. It persists (*chronicum*) and slowly expands (*migrans*). Some 25 per cent of cases do not recall getting a tick bite or ECM. Stage 2 is marked by fever, headache, chills, muscular aches and joint pains. These are often intermittent, but fatigue and malaise are constant and may be debilitating. Once again you can see that it resembles CFS in many respects, and may be confused with it. Sometimes the central nervous system or other vital organs are affected in Lyme disease (in which case meningitis or varying degrees of paralysis may occur). These are not likely to be confused with CFS. Stage 3 occurs in up to 60 per cent of cases many months after the initial infection. The typical picture is one of a relapsing remitting arthritis.

Glandular fever

Glandular fever is a well-known viral illness. If we come across the culprit virus in early childhood, we may never even know we had it. Young children may experience a slight sore throat or may have no symptoms at all (so called subclinical infection). In adolescents the classical features of sore throat, swollen glands, fatigue, malaise and fever are more common. In severe cases the liver, spleen and heart can be affected, but most patients get over the infection within four to six weeks. However, fatigue and poor concentration may persist for many months. In a small percentage of cases the blood test for glandular fever remains positive for a very long time, and may be associated with chronic debilitating fatigue.

Cytomegalovirus

A cytomegalovirus infection in an otherwise healthy adult can produce an illness very similar to glandular fever (they're both called infectious mononeucleosis) except that it rarely produces a sore throat and swollen glands in the neck. Most patients recover after four to six weeks, but postviral fatigue and weakness may persist for many months.

Polio virus

Polio outbreaks are much less common since the advent of immunisation, but they still occur from time to time, even in well-immunised communities. Up to 40 per cent of polio survivors develop a state of chronic debilitating fatigue some twenty-five to thirty-five years after apparent recovery. In other words, they get over the initial bout of polio and lead virtually normal lives for several decades. Then they decline into a postpolio syndrome, characterised by fatigue, muscular weakness, aches and pains, and cold intolerance. Some of them become very debilitated. That's the bad news. The good news is that the condition is only very slowly progressive, and that 91 per cent of patients can be stabilised by simple measures: simplify work, conserve energy and reduce stress. The postpolio syndrome is perhaps unique in this regard. All other fatigued patients are encouraged to gradually increase their daily activities and to follow a prescribed exercise programme; postpolio patients should only do so with great caution and under medical supervision.

Other candidates

There are of course whole stables of infectious agents that can cause similar problems, namely, an acute illness (with occasional complications) followed by complete recovery, but resulting in persistent fatigue in a minority of unfortunate individuals. If the fatigue endures beyond six months, a diagnosis of post-infectious or postviral fatigue syndrome (PVFS) should be considered. These are subgroups of CFS and should be treated as such. Remember, at this stage it does not matter what the original bug was. If you were in good health until you contracted an infection, whatever the infection, and have not felt well since, you should seriously consider a diagnosis of CFS.

Multiple Chemical Sensitivity Syndrome

20

Man has introduced countless chemicals to his environment since the Industrial Revolution, and continues to add to the tally at a present rate of 1,000 new compounds each year. At least 10,000 of these are in regular use. Each one of us will encounter an estimated 200 man-made chemicals during the course of a normal day, and up to 400 if we live or work in a chemically laden environment. This proliferation of chemical use is now an issue of environmental concern. We have indiscriminately thrown thousands of tons of chemical waste into our water, soil and air.

On a global scale, we have punched a hole in the ozone layer; and at national level, we find many countries in dire straits with uncontrolled pollution. We must not believe for one moment that we can inflict such damage on our environment without incurring some penalty on health. After all, we are an integral part of the environment. We eat the food, drink the water and breathe the air. In so doing, and if I may borrow a phrase, we *internalise* the environment we live in.

We should not think, therefore, in terms of the 'environment' and 'us', but in terms of our external and internal environments as a continuum. We cannot expect to harm one without also harming the other. For example, during the past twenty years industrialised countries have witnessed an alarming rise in allergic diseases, and air pollution may be a significant contributing factor in this.

Many pollutants build up in our bodies over time. For instance, PCBs (polychlorinated biphenyls), widely used in the electrical industry, have been detected in the breast milk of nursing mothers. They are thought to contribute to increased rates of infection in the newborn. Likewise, pollutants have been detected in our blood, sweat and urine. There can be little doubt then that we are collectively affected by what we throw into our environment.

We also hear of individuals being poisoned in various ways by toxic chemicals — chemical warfare, commercial negligence, occupational and domestic accidents all occur. We have heard of the Gulf War syndrome, for example, a debilitating condition affecting many veterans of Desert Storm. It is thought to have been caused, at least in part, by chemical exposures suffered by soldiers during their tour of duty in the Persian Gulf. Negligent exposures are also well publicised, for example, the outbreak of illness among seventy people who ate cucumber contaminated with pesticide. In contrast, occupational and domestic accidents receive less attention. The farmer who falls into a sheep dip, or the gardener who sprays himself with herbicide, is not going to make it into the news. As you will see, these poisonings may lead to very troublesome illnesses.

Before we proceed, I should mention the other ways in which chemicals are known to affect individual health.

1. Allergic reactions to chemicals may be implicated as a trigger in many conditions, including contact allergic dermatitis, conjunctivitis, rhinitis, asthma, urticaria and anaphylaxis.
2. Irritant reactions to chemicals may also contribute to or exacerbate these disorders.
3. Intolerant reactions to chemicals may exacerbate some cases of hyperactivity and migraine.

In summary, then, we have established that chemicals may give rise to pollutant, toxic, allergic, intolerant and irritant effects. In this chapter, however, I want to address something quite different; I want to talk about canaries!

Case history

Rory was a farmer who kept livestock. One day, as he was inspecting his herd, a dreadful accident occurred. A plane, which had strayed off course, flew overhead and doused him with pesticide. He suffered the immediate effects of chemical toxicity, and ran back to his house for a shower. By the time he got there, his eyes were red and sore, his nose was burning, and he developed a hacking painful cough. Some of these symptoms settled after a wash and a change of clothes, but other symptoms soon took their place. His head was pounding, he felt nauseous and his muscles started to twitch. He was admitted to hospital. Although his acute symptoms settled down after a few days, he was left feeling very tired and ill. That was twenty years ago, and Rory has never felt well since. His doctors had no difficulty diagnosing his original illness: he had acute organophosphate poisoning, but they found it more difficult to understand the vague and chronic symptoms which he experienced subsequently. For instance, every time he got a whiff of paint he collapsed to the ground — just fell like a ton of bricks! Sometimes he would start to shake uncontrollably with muscle spasms. His doctor was called to the scene on more than one occasion to provide emergency treatment. Over the years, Rory started to react in this way to a host of other smells, including perfumes, air fresheners, traffic fumes and the like. This forced him to adopt a secluded lifestyle, for he could not bear to collapse in front of his perfumed (or aftershaved) friends. Rory has multiple chemical sensitivity — he's a canary!

In times past, miners took canaries down their shafts, and kept them in cages close to the coal face. Their reason for doing so was simple, if somewhat cruel. Miners were at risk of poisoning from dangerous gases emanating from the coal face, and they had no way of knowing when the levels were high. Canaries, being very sensitive creatures, react swiftly to changes in their environment. They die in the presence of *relatively low amounts* of toxic gas. A dead canary was a sign to the miners that they too were at risk of poisoning, and that they should leave the mine post-haste. Rory, and others like him, are sensitive to relatively low amounts of environmental chemicals, much lower levels than would be required to cause visible signs of poisoning. These chemically sensitive canaries, by their suffering, may be sending a warning signal to the rest of us: clean up your act; think again about these chemicals; you cannot afford to pollute your environment.

You may find all this a little hard to believe. After all, you may say, we are talking about polish and perfume. Surely they can't make you ill! Moreover, you may confidently cite the safety declarations of our public health officials. They tell us reassuringly that the chemicals in common use are safe, and that, as long as we take precautions, even the more toxic chemicals can be used without harmful effects. This is of course true — in so far as it goes. The same scientists, however, will readily admit that their statements refer only to toxicity, and not to issues of individual sensitivity. They can tell us, for example, that a particular chemical is either poisonous or safe, and that it will or it won't cause cancer. When dealing with shades of grey, they can tell us at what dose a safe chemical becomes poisonous. Their confidence is based on the fact that the toxic effect of chemicals can be easily measured. In stark contrast, the subjective claims of chemical sensitivity are much more difficult to assess. They do not lend themselves to the same scrutiny. Similarly, it is difficult to assess the health effects of prolonged exposure to low doses of chemical, or to mixtures of chemicals. The hardy (miners) among us may not be unduly worried about this, but the sensitive (canaries) most certainly are.

Aoife's story

I should know a little bit about canaries; I married one! And I would like, at this point, to relate a very personal story. It is one which has changed my life in many ways and for obvious reasons. It has also changed my whole approach to the practice of medicine, in that it introduced me to the exciting new field of allergy and environmental medicine. My wife, Aoife, had always been an energetic sort of person who enjoyed excellent health. She had an avid interest in people with whom she would spend hours on end in animated conversation. In the earlier years of our marriage we had frequent moves (to facilitate my postgraduate training). At one stage we lived in a small but beautiful lodge. It was heated by a twenty-year-old oil burner which was situated in the kitchen and which constantly smelt of oil. The smell was faint and we soon grew used to it. After ten months in this little house, Aoife gradually lost her appetite, felt nauseated and became uncharacteristically tired.

The nausea was unresponsive to the usual medication, so she was admitted to hospital for investigation. An endoscope (internal telescope) revealed that she had gastritis (an inflamed stomach) and she was treated appropriately. However, the nausea and fatigue continued in spite of treatment and in spite of the fact that a repeat endoscopy showed healing to be well under way.

We then moved house again, this time into a cramped hospital flat, in which we relied on a gas cooker for all our meals. Some six months later, whilst still nauseated and fatigued, Aoife suddenly developed a piercing headache which affected the right side of her head and her right eye. The nausea worsened and she started to vomit. Two days into the headache she complained of a sensation of pins and needles and, subsequently, of a loss of power in her right arm and leg — she had a partial paralysis on the right-hand side of her body (hemiplegia). A brain tumour was suspected, so she was admitted to a neurosurgical ward for investigation. Fortunately, no tumour was found, and a diagnosis of hemiplegic migraine was eventually made. The standard medical treatment for migraine failed to relieve either the severity or frequency of the migraine attacks.

It is difficult to describe the sheer agony of the next four years. Aoife was practically house-bound, and often bed-bound. She felt utterly exhausted, and she had (by now) a permanent headache which was interspersed with severe hemiplegic migraine attacks. She became so depressed that she considered suicide — it seemed the only escape from unrelenting pain. I carried on as best I could in training, and later in general practice. You can imagine my despair and frustration at not being able to help my own wife. The sad truth is that the entire resources of my profession were unable to relieve her suffering — day after day, for four years, fatigue, headache, nausea, vomiting, weakness. I disconnected the doorbell, switched off the phone and put a 'DO NOT DISTURB' sign on the front door. Inside, Aoife kept the curtains closed to shut out the light. Noise and light were painful. The animated conversation had long since ceased — she could hardly manage the social niceties, let alone engage in meaningful chat. She did manage, on her better days, to get out and about, but she would never make a social promise, as she knew not from one day to the next whether she would be well enough to keep it.

In desperation, I turned to a consultant physician with an interest in allergy and environmental medicine, Dr Ronald Finn of the Royal Liverpool Hospital. I displayed my complete ignorance by asking the question: 'Do you think her illness might have anything to do with food?' Dr Finn saw Aoife and put her through the paces of a low allergy diet. Within two days, she experienced flu-like aches and pains and the headache worsened. At first I was puzzled, and then ecstatic when Dr Finn told me that these were classical withdrawal symptoms, and she must therefore have had hidden food intolerance. However, by the seventh day there was no improvement: the fatigue, nausea and headache continued unabated. She then restricted her diet to lamb and pear for ten days, and then a total fast for five days, but to no avail. In the meantime, I read a book recommended to me by Dr Finn entitled *The Migraine Revolution* (Thorsons), written by Dr John Mansfield. He described how migraine can be sometimes caused not only by foods, but by sensitivity to domestic chemicals (such as gas or oil fumes), and that in certain cases both food and chemicals are involved simultaneously

Having had no success on the dietary side, we turned our attention to chemicals and organised a chemical-free holiday for Aoife. She went to stay with friends who lived in an all-electric house. Within five days she had made a remarkable recovery: the headache was gone, the nausea had cleared and her energy returned — for the first time in four years. I still have a vivid memory of the smile on her face when I came to collect her at the weekend. She had found relief at last!

The symptoms flared up again within four days of returning home, so we turned off the gas at the mains, and the symptoms gradually subsided over the following week. The doorbell was reconnected, the phone allowed to ring, and the 'DO NOT DISTURB' sign was unceremoniously dumped in the bin! A neighbour commented that the curtains were no longer constantly closed, and that the sound of lively chat was heard once more in our house.

Apart from enjoying an enormous improvement in health, Aoife felt somewhat vindicated by her recovery. However loyal they may be, it is hard for friends to appreciate how ill you are when you have nothing to show for your illness. They may even doubt that you are ill at all, and this — together with accusations of hysteria which may be levelled at you by some doctors (as they were at Aoife) — can leave you feeling very lonely indeed.

We now live in an all-electric house. The central heating is provided by an oil-fired burner situated in a *separate* building (a shed in the back garden) to ensure that no oil fumes accumulate inside the house. Aoife has remained well since then. She has had no hemiplegic migraine, and the awful fatigue is a thing of the past. For the sake of completeness, I should say that Aoife did experience some return of headache in each postnatal period, and that she is prone to headache when she is sleep deprived, but these headaches are nothing when compared to the previous ones. We later discovered a number of culprit foods which were contributing to her headaches (this explains why she had withdrawal symptoms on the low allergy diet without the anticipated improvement — the benefit of the wash-out was completely swept aside by her ongoing exposure to gas fumes). Furthermore, whenever Aoife is exposed to gas fumes, she develops nausea, dots before the eyes, fatigue and — unless she escapes — headache. We shall be forever grateful to Drs Finn and Mansfield for their help.

What is multiple chemical sensitivity?

Multiple chemical sensitivity (MCS) is a term used to describe patients who have hypersensitive reactions to many otherwise harmless chemicals. They also react to toxic chemicals at very low doses, far below those expected to cause symptoms in the general population. Many of these patients give a clear history of a single poisonous exposure from which they have never recovered; others develop the problem after prolonged exposure to lower, non-poisonous levels of chemical. In all cases, patients are left with an extreme sensitivity to ordinary chemical smells, including perfume, aftershave, deodorants, hair gel, make-up, air fresheners, tobacco smoke, exhaust fumes, newspaper print, new fabric, new cars, photocopiers, printers and plastics. The symptoms they complain of are numerous and include:

- Fatigue
- Headache (including migraine)
- Nausea
- Depression and irritability
- Mood swings
- Anxiety
- Impaired memory and concentration
- Pains in the muscles and joints
- Sleep complaints.

In addition, some of these patients have

- Increased heart rate
- High blood pressure
- Increased breathing rate (overbreathing)
- Symptoms of food intolerance (see below).

Who gets it?

We have no way of predicting who will become chemically sensitive. It is said to be more common in women, but this difference may be slight. Acute poisoning with toxic chemicals, or prolonged exposure to less toxic chemicals, are definite risk factors; and, indeed, these 'sensitising' events are essential prerequisites for the disorder. However, not all poisoned patients will develop chemical sensitivity. This suggests that other factors, as yet unknown, increase the risk for some individuals.

Will they grow out of it?

Chemical poisoning, if severe, can lead to permanent health problems in its own right. These are the direct effects of toxicity and they should be distinguished from the symptoms of sensitivity (which may or may not develop after the poisoning). Once they have been sensitised, these patients are likely to retain their sensitivity throughout their lives. However, with proper care and treatment many patients can enjoy significant relief.

What causes it?

We are not yet sure of the cause of chemical sensitivity. However, we know that chemical poisoning frequently and seriously disrupts nerve pathways in the brain. Furthermore, we recognise that many of the symptoms of the syndrome, including depression and anxiety, are also *the result of brain dysfunction*. This leads us to a very interesting and plausible theory. It goes something like this:

1. There is an initial exposure to chemicals. This may be either sudden or gradual.
2. The chemicals are transported to the brain via the olfactory (smell) nerve, and/or the bloodstream.
3. Susceptible people cannot cope with the chemical onslaught.
4. Their brain becomes saturated or overloaded with chemical.
5. Nerve pathways in the brain become sensitised to chemicals. They lose their previous tolerance, and they develop hypersensitive responses to everyday low-level chemical exposures. They react even to chemicals which are unrelated to the initial exposure.
6. Their brain is left in a state of persistent hypersensitivity, and symptoms arise from the disruption that ensues.
7. Many of the symptoms can be understood in terms of the particular parts of the brain that are affected, including the symptoms of depression and anxiety.

This theory is referred to as neurosensitisation, or time-dependent sensitisation. In most cases, the initial exposure is sudden and poisonous, frequently requiring emergency medical treatment; in other cases, the exposure is much more gradual and subtle.

Case history

Mark had worked in the family business all his life. He owned a petrol station and fixed cars, and did so with impunity for many years. However, he developed symptoms in his late thirties, namely, headaches, pains in his eyes, sore muscles, general tiredness and 'terrible indigestion'. By now his symptoms were very disabling, and his life had become miserable. In fact, he was downright cranky, his sleep was disturbed and unrefreshing, and his concentration was at an all-time low. As he related the story, he gave one interesting clue: his symptoms improved away from work. This could be the simple benefit of rest, of course, but it could equally signify a chemical sensitivity. Mark was advised to go on a 'chemical holiday' (see page 282). His symptoms improved dramatically during this time. We then organised a phased return to work, being careful to limit his exposure to chemicals. He discovered that he could work in the shop all day and run the business from there without symptoms. However, his symptoms returned as soon as he started to fill petrol. He had developed chemical sensitivity after many years of low-dose exposure to petrochemical fumes.

Are there any complications?

The lives of chemically sensitive patients are severely disrupted by their need to avoid chemical smells. Moreover, they have a financial burden to bear, in that as many as 70 per cent give up their jobs on account of the illness. They may also run into trouble with their family and friends, who find it difficult to understand this puzzling and controversial disorder. In addition, chemical sensitivity is frequently complicated by food intolerance.

Case history

Consider Abigail, for instance, a 32-year-old scientist. She was working in the research and development department of a multinational firm. One day there was a chemical spillage in her laboratory and she became violently ill. She was admitted to hospital with headache, nausea and muscle pains. That was a year ago, and she has suffered ever since. In particular, she complained of fatigue, depression, anxiety, headaches and muscle spasms. She also developed asthma and rhinitis. Some of her symptoms got worse when she was exposed to chemical smells — even smells we take for granted, such as pot-pourri and perfumed soap.

By the time she presented to the allergy clinic, several hospital specialists had reassured her that nothing physical was wrong. By this they meant that they could find no physical explanation for her symptoms. She did not have a brain tumour, her blood was healthy and she had no obvious signs of disease. She was told that her symptoms were 'functional', in other words, everything *looked* OK; it just didn't *function* properly.

Antidepressant medication improved her mental state considerably, but she was left with her most troublesome symptoms. Having thus excluded any other explanation for her symptoms, and in some desperation, Abigail went on a ten day low allergy diet. To her great relief, all her symptoms improved. She identified the problem foods one by one, and remains well as long as she avoids these. She is also careful to avoid chemical smells, but even these are more easily coped with now that she is eating the right diet. Abigail had multiple chemical sensitivity, but most of her symptoms were due to the associated food intolerance.

This case raises another important issue, namely, the concept of 'total load'. Let me explain. Abigail had a poisonous event from which she developed chemical sensitivity. This in turn led to food intolerance. Thus, she was reacting adversely to many chemicals and, although she didn't know it at the time, several foods. The total load on her system was considerable. When she reduced the load (by avoiding intolerant foods and chemical smells), she was much better able to cope with transient chemical exposures.

There is nothing particularly unusual about Abigail. Doctors working in environmental medicine have long observed the clinical association between chemical sensitivity, food intolerance, chronic fatigue and type 1 allergies. This led one author (Dr C. S. Miller) to propose a new theory of disease, namely, toxicant-induced loss of tolerance — TILT. The theory posits that single high-dose chemical exposures, or repeated low-dose exposures, can lead to a general loss of tolerance to chemicals, foods and other allergens.

What can we do about it?

If you suspect that you are suffering from chemical sensitivity, go on a 'chemical holiday' (see page 282). The best treatment for chemical sensitivity is avoidance of chemical smells. In fact, therein lies a good rule of thumb: if it smells, avoid it! Reduce your total load by the following means:

1. Create a home which is free of chemicals.
   - See 'Advice for the chemically sensitive' (pages 209–10).
2. Tell your friends.
   - They will need to be aware of the problem if they're to avoid polluting the environment that you have spent so long cleaning up.
3. Check out your other sensitivities.
   - All patients with multiple chemical sensitivity should consider the low allergy diet for food intolerance (see Chapter 15).
   - They should also consider the possibility of gut fermentation (see page 177).
4. Consider a course of desensitisation which works well for many patients (see Appendix 1).

Could it be anything else?

Multiple chemical sensitivity is said by some to be a psychiatric disorder. They base their assertion on the fact that the condition defies all the established doctrines of toxicology. They point out that none of these patients has 'tissue pathology' or other visible effects of toxic poisoning. They also remind us that many of these patients are depressed and anxious. However, I trust that these arguments have been adequately addressed in the text above.

There are, of course, occasional patients who wrongly attribute their symptoms to chemical sensitivity. Take the social phobic, for example. She doesn't want to meet people. She's too shy. It is much easier for her to say, 'I cannot go out because I have MCS', than admit to her real pain. Meeting people makes her feel terribly inadequate. She has very low self-esteem and doesn't want to be reminded of it. In the same vein, the depressed man may be unhappy or anxious for any number of reasons, but he has learned that men are macho, men don't cry, and men certainly cannot admit to psychological weakness. It is much easier for him to complain to his doctor about physical symptoms than emotional ones.

The assessment of any patient with suspected multiple chemical sensitivity must, therefore, be compassionate and dispassionate all at once. It is wrong to tell patients that their symptoms are physical in origin when they are in fact psychological.

Advice for the chemically sensitive

1. You will need to recruit the co-operation of all household members to achieve a low-chemical environment.
   - Beware of teenagers who spray themselves in their bedrooms — the fumes will travel.

2. Do not use cosmetics, especially if they are perfumed.
   - Use lemon juice as an astringent.
   - Use olive or baby oil as a cleansing cream.
   - Use peeled and sliced cucumber puréed with one teaspoon of yoghurt as a freshener.
   - Make up a moisturising cream as follows: one tablespoon each of honey, water and olive oil, mixed with one capsule of vitamin E.
   - You may get away with unperfumed hypo-allergenic cosmetics.
   - You might also get away with a baby shampoo.
   - Use unscented stick deodorants.

3. Minimise your exposure to soaps, polishes, bleach etc.
   - Use baking soda or borax as an all-purpose cleaner.
   - Wash windows with vinegar (one tablespoon) in water (a half-pint).
   - Clean the fridge with soda water.
   - Dust with a damp cloth.
   - Polish with beeswax.

4. Do not use air fresheners.
   - Use vinegar or baking soda in water. Leave it sitting in a saucer in a corner of the room.

5. You will also need to be aware of other chemical sources.
   - Gas fires and cookers, for example, are heavy contaminants. Electric ones are better.

6. Similarly, the central heating boiler may leak tiny amounts of fumes into the atmosphere.
   - Boilers are better housed in a separate building, such as a

shed in the back garden.
- Leave a few feet of fresh air between the flue and your main dwelling.
- If you have an integral garage, seal the communicating door.

7. Check out your car.
    - Get rid of your old car if it smells of petrol or diesel.
    - Don't buy a new car, they're too smelly. Go for something six to twelve months old.
    - Saloons are better than hatchbacks.

Section 4

Chronic Debilitating Fatigue

21 *Fibromyalgia*

Also sometimes called non-specific rheumatism or muscular rheumatism

Case history

Jane is a 50-year-old mother of two who helps to run the family retail business. She is busy, but she enjoys her lifestyle. She was increasingly frustrated by her lack of health, and in particular she complained of generalised aches and pains. These became quite severe at times, and would force her to stop whatever she was doing. They also prevented her from getting to sleep and frequently woke her out of sleep in the dead of night. She had pain in her arms and legs, her back and her chest. Her neck and scalp were also sore and she had frequent headaches. She was embarrassed to tell me that she could not allow her husband to hold her, as she was so tender. Her sex life was therefore non-existent.

She was also tired all the time and prone to bouts of depression. Finally, her bowel was acting up with many of the symptoms of an irritable bowel syndrome. As time went by she was more and more restricted in terms of what she could achieve. She tried many different medical treatments, but none of these gave her the relief she needed. Her energy was now fading and unreliable, lifting aggravated her pain, and she could never stray too far from the toilet in case of urgent need. Her doctor referred her to the allergy clinic.

Jane was unable to tell me when she last felt perfectly well. She had had pains for as long as she could remember, even as far back as childhood. That in itself was interesting and prompted a low allergy diet. Two weeks later, Jane reported that she had classical withdrawal symptoms for the first four days, followed by better quality sleep, more energy and a general reduction in pain. She had no symptoms of an irritable bowel. Her diet was then expanded into relatively safe areas (foods that are least likely to cause intolerant reactions) and she continued to improve over the following month. She was now left with pain in the arms; all other pains had ceased. A closer look at this persistent pain revealed that it was probably coming from her neck and she was referred to physiotherapy for treatment of this. Jane had fibromyalgia, and in her case it was related to diet. She should do very well with treatment.

What is fibromyalgia?

Fibromyalgia is a disorder that affects up to 4 per cent of the general population. It is more common in women. The cardinal symptom is widespread pain, with areas of local tenderness. In this context, there is a difference between pain and tenderness. Pain has a life of its own. It comes on without being evoked. Tenderness, on the other hand, refers to pain evoked by touch. Once again we have diagnostic criteria to help us identify symptom clusters. Strictly speaking, to meet the diagnostic criteria for fibromyalgia, digital palpation with an approximate force of 4 kg must produce a report of pain in at least eleven of eighteen recognised points. These points are listed below. For the sake of accuracy I have used medical terminology here, but explanations appear in parentheses, and a diagram is provided for the sake of clarity.

1. Suboccipital muscle insertions at occiput (where the neck muscles insert at the base of the skull, on either side).
2. Lower cervical paraspinals (where the shoulder and neck muscles meet).
3. Trapezius at midpoint of the upper border (midway between the base of the neck and the shoulder tip).
4. Supraspinatus at its origin above medial scapular spine (on the wing bone).
5. Second costochondral junction (where the second rib joins the breast plate).

6. Two centimetres distal to lateral epicondyle in forearm (just below the outer aspect of the elbow).
7. Upper outer quadrant of buttock.
8. Greater trochanter (the hip bone).
9. Knee just proximal to the medial joint line (just above the inner aspect of the knee).

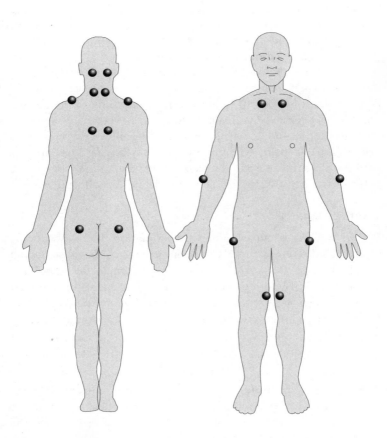

The tenderness at these sites should be focal rather than diffuse, i.e. at the site of pressure only. Tenderness may be present at other sites also. Additional requirements for the diagnosis are:

- Tender points must be present on both sides of the body.
- Tender points must be present above and below the waist.
- Widespread pain must have been present for at least three months.

A number of other symptoms may be present in addition to pain. These include marked fatigue, morning stiffness, sleep disturbance and headache. Some doctors will accept a diagnosis of fibromyalgia with fewer than eleven tender points, if several of these associated symptoms are also present.

The fatigue that accompanies fibromyalgia is profound; so much so that it may be confused with the fatigue of a chronic fatigue syndrome (CFS). Although the symptoms of these two conditions overlap significantly, they are nevertheless separate and distinct entities. Simply put, the dominant symptom in fibromyalgia is pain, whereas in CFS it's fatigue. Fibromyalgia patients will say, 'Get rid of my pain. I can live with the fatigue.' CFS patients will say, 'Get rid of my fatigue. I can live with the pain.'

What causes it?

We do not know what causes the condition, but we strongly suspect that sleep disruption is an important contributing factor, particularly in the early days of onset. Once the condition becomes established, it can be difficult to shift, even after a regular sleep pattern is secured. I have seen many patients with fibromyalgia who could trace the onset of their trouble to sleep deprivation.

Case history

Paula, for example, was a 29-year-old housewife who complained of 'general tenderness in the bones'. She was also lacking in energy. Her symptoms had been present since the birth of her third child, a boy now aged 5 years. Significantly, her sleep was badly disrupted by the new arrival. At first, the pains were only affecting one joint at a time. Then they flitted around from one joint to the next. After some time, and in spite of several visits to the doctor, her symptoms became worse. She was now quite stiff in the mornings and her muscles were sore to touch. She could not stand being bumped into in a crowd. Nor could she endure being hugged. She was sore all over and, at this stage, quite miserable with the whole affair. The young lad was now sleeping through the night, but Paula was still tossing and turning restlessly. She had developed fibromyalgia and she had no problem believing that her sleep, or the lack of it, had contributed to her symptoms.

As it happens, Paula, like Jane, embarked on a low allergy diet which improved the quality of her sleep. Her hands were not as stiff or painful, and the awful 'sore all over' feeling was much less than previously. Food challenges were then given, one by one, until she had identified all her safe foods, as well as a few that disrupted her sleep. She now avoids these foods and remains well. Symptoms are apt to return if her sleep is disrupted for any reason.

How interesting, don't you think? Both Jane and Paula enjoyed better quality sleep on the low allergy diet. I strongly suspect that this was the mechanism by which their fibromyalgia improved.

More controversy

Fibromyalgia, like CFS, is a taboo subject in the minds of some conventional doctors. This is so because fibromyalgia, like CFS, is a clinical diagnosis (made on the grounds of the pattern of symptoms only), and because pain, like fatigue, cannot be measured objectively or confirmed by laboratory investigations. Furthermore, depression and anxiety often complicate the clinical picture of fibromyalgia, and this has led some to suggest that it is really a 'psychogenic rheumatism' — in much the same way that CFS is said to be 'just another form of depression'. However, and for those who will take the time to read them, several studies have established that fibromyalgia is neither psychosomatic nor hysterical in origin. Anxiety and depression, when present (because they are not always so), are likely to be the result rather than the cause of these disabling disorders.

What can we do about it?

The principles of treatment for fibromyalgia are very similar to the treatment of CFS and other states of debilitating fatigue of unknown origin. These are outlined in Chapter 25.

22   *Chronic Fatigue Syndrome*

This condition is also referred to as postviral fatigue syndrome (PVFS) and myalgic encephalomyelitis (ME).

Case history

John first became ill when he was 25 years old. Until then he had enjoyed excellent physical and mental health. He was a keen and competitive athlete, but he had not overtrained; nor had he taken steroids (both of which could have induced fatigue). He was also a successful salesman. He held one of the best work performance records in his company and was being considered for promotion. He enjoyed his work, his marriage, and a diverse social life.

Then one day he suddenly became ill with a high fever, headache, lethargy and severe chest pains. He quickly developed pneumonia, became increasingly short of breath and was admitted to the intensive care unit in a critical state. He was told that he had Bornholm disease, a viral infection renowned for its propensity to cause muscle pain and which may sometimes cause meningitis, as it did in his case. Although he was well enough to be discharged from hospital shortly afterwards, he never recovered his full strength. Indeed, he was a mere shadow of his former self.

His family doctor had no idea what was wrong with him and sent him to see a psychiatrist. The psychiatrist ignored his precipitating illness, told him that he was depressed and gave him an antidepressant. This did not help him at all.

When he first came to see me some three years later, he was still feeling tired all the time. He complained of being uncharacteristically irritable and of having constant pain in his chest and leg muscles. He said that his sleep was disturbed by 'an overactive mind', that his concentration was poor, and that he was feeling rather low in himself. All his symptoms were made worse by exertion, and relieved somewhat — but only somewhat — by rest. With this in mind, he took a six week holiday in quest of relief, but to no avail.

In spite of his debilitating symptoms, he has worked hard to maintain his position in the company. To this end, he has pushed himself to the limit and is, by now, utterly exhausted. At the end of a day at work, he returns to his wife and home, collapses in a soft chair and tries to relax. He wants to be left there undisturbed to recover whatever strength he can for the next gruelling day. Alone with his feelings, he wonders whether he will ever get better again, and he feels increasingly frustrated by the limitations imposed upon him by this dreaded illness. John has chronic fatigue syndrome.

What is chronic fatigue syndrome?

Chronic fatigue syndrome (CFS) is a state of persistent and debilitating fatigue of unknown origin. The most widely adopted definition of CFS is the one proposed by Fukuda and colleagues at the Centre for Disease Control (Atlanta, USA) in 1994. They characterise chronic fatigue syndrome as follows:

Criterion A

	Yes/No
• A state of persistent or relapsing debilitating fatigue which is of new or definite onset, which has been fully evaluated clinically, and which cannot be otherwise explained, and which	
• has been present for six months or longer,	
• is not substantially relieved by rest,	
• is not the result of ongoing exertion, and	
• results in substantial reductions in previous levels of occupational, social, personal or educational activity.	

In addition, there is a requirement for the new and concurrent presence of four or more of the following symptoms during six consecutive months of illness:

Criterion B

Yes/No

	Yes/No
• impairment of short-term memory or concentration	
• sore throats	
• tender lymph glands (in the neck or axillae)	
• muscle pains	
• joint pains (without redness or swelling)	
• headaches (new in type, pattern or severity)	
• unrefreshing sleep	
• post-exertional malaise (in excess of 24 hours' duration)	

If you have answered yes to all five points of criterion A, and to four or more of the criterion B symptoms, you may have CFS. Read on.

It stands to reason that these (criterion B) symptoms, like the fatigue they accompany, should also be of new onset. Thus the joint pains of pre-existing arthritis, or the headache of a patient with a history of migraine, should not count in a diagnosis of CFS. However, if the joint pains or headache etc. are of new severity or quality, then they are taken into account. Similarly, we do *not* diagnose CFS in those who have

1. other medical explanations for their fatigue, such as a low blood count, hypothyroidism etc.
2. a past or current diagnosis of psychotic depression, manic depression, schizophrenia, delusional disorders, dementia, anorexia nervosa or bulimia nervosa.
3. a history of alcohol or substance abuse two years prior to the onset of their fatigue, or at any other time thereafter.
4. a problem with severe obesity (a BMI greater than, or equal to 45).

Before the discerning reader objects, let me acknowledge that these diagnostic criteria are fallible. Who, for example, is to say that one patient does not have CFS because they have been ill for just under six months, and to another that they have because they have been ill for six months and a day? Similarly, we acknowledge from the outset that this arbitrary definition will exclude those who have less severe or less typical forms of the illness. Furthermore, patients with psychiatric disorders are not immune from allergies, infections, cancer, or any other disease for that matter. Who then can deny them the right to develop a chronic fatigue syndrome? Nevertheless, these strict criteria serve several important functions. Firstly, they ensure that those who do have exclusionary disorders are identified as such and treated with appropriate medical care. Secondly, they enable us to identify, with at least some degree of international consistency, a group of patients whose lives are significantly affected by chronic debilitating fatigue. Such homogeneity provides us with both research and clinical benefits. It would be well nigh impossible to research CFS if we allowed it to be diluted with the pathologies of other disorders. Studying 'pure' CFS, on the other hand, gives our research efforts the best possible chance of a break-through. Homogeneity also provides us with an opportunity to develop clinical expertise in dealing with individual patients and in helping them to manage their condition.

We also refer to non-exclusionary disorders. These are symptoms that may occur before, during or after the onset of CFS, that are not part of the definition of CFS *per se*, but which do not preclude the diagnosis of CFS. These include anxiety, depression, somatisation, fibromyalgia and multiple chemical sensitivity, among others.

I must confess that I have a bone to pick here. It is my personal belief that somatisation should be considered an exclusionary disorder for CFS. You will recall from our previous discussion that the somatisation disorders may involve some degree of gain for the patient. The primary gain is the immediate relief of psychological distress (by converting it to physical sensations), and the secondary gains are variable. Thus, somatisation is far too complex a psychological problem to allow it to co-exist with CFS — an already complex illness. To do so would be to complicate the clinical picture enormously. At the very least, patients who fulfil the diagnostic criteria for CFS *and* somatisation should be clearly distinguished from patients who have CFS alone. Why? Because patients with CFS and somatisation have higher rates of psychiatric illness and longer illness duration than those who have CFS alone. This is hardly surprising, for we saw that 90 per cent of somatisers are still stuck in their unhappy state ten years later. Furthermore, the 1988 definition which preceded the current one was criticised because it included too many physical symptoms and tended to 'pick up' somatisers.

How does CFS start?

The typical patient will say: 'I was in perfect health until I came down with a virus some time ago, and I've never been well since.' When asked for more details of their initial illness, they describe the universal symptoms of an acute viral infection, such as high fever, headache, muscle pains and extreme lethargy. In addition, the signature symptoms of the offending virus are also present. Thus, the Epstein-Barr virus causes glandular fever (sore throat and swollen glands); the Coxsackie viruses cause Bornholm disease (severe chest pains); the influenza viruses give rise to respiratory symptoms, and so on. The patient will usually have been confined to bed in the early stages of his illness.

Whereas the vast majority of us recover well and without incident from such infections within a matter of days or weeks, a few unfortunate people do not. The latter may feel somewhat better shortly after they first become ill, but they suddenly get worse again with a return of all their old symptoms: headache, muscle pain, sore throat and fatigue etc. They may now enter a period of prolonged debility. Anything less than six months in duration is called postviral debility; anything beyond that is referred to as a chronic fatigue syndrome. There are several good reasons for this arbitrary six month cut-off point. In the first place, fatigue may be the presenting feature of virtually any disease, so we allow time for other symptoms to develop — other clues, as it were, that may lead to a specific diagnosis. Secondly, postviral debility is common in otherwise healthy individuals. A good bout of flu, for example, can take six weeks to get over, and debility extending beyond that is quite possible. But for every one hundred patients who are still debilitated at, say, the four month mark, only one will remain ill and qualify for a diagnosis of CFS.

Eighty per cent of all cases of CFS start in this manner, in the immediate aftermath of an infection. The terms 'postinfectious' or 'postviral fatigue syndrome' are therefore sometimes used for these. The remaining 20 per cent of cases are indistinguishable in terms of their symptoms, the only difference being an inability to recall a precipitating infectious illness. Some of these may start shortly after an operation, an accident, or some other major adverse life event, such as bereavement. In fact, in one study, 85 per cent of all patients with CFS had experienced significant stress in the year leading up to their illness. This would include patients who became ill after an infection. We can understand this in the light of our knowledge that stress can lower immunity and affect our ability to handle infection. We also know that stress, especially if prolonged, has a direct adverse effect on the brain, and specifically on the HPA axis (see page 243).

Half of my own patients admit to stress in the lead-up to their CFS. The stressors identified include work or study-related stress, frequent travel, moving house, bereavement and financial anxiety, among others.

Who gets it?

Anyone can get CFS, although we do not like to diagnose it in very young children. My oldest patient was an 83-year-old woman, my youngest a 9-year-old boy, both of whom made excellent recoveries (and neither of whom could be described as yuppies). Furthermore, cases of CFS can be found wherever they are sought (irrespective of gender, social class, nationality, personality type etc.) at the rate of approximately one per 1,000 population. This figure is remarkably consistent internationally, which suggests the involvement of a definite genetic element. Patients with a previous history of major depression are thought to be at increased risk, as are patients who experience significant viral infections such as glandular fever, Q fever, cytomegalovirus etc. Common infective episodes, on the other hand, are not a risk factor.

Controversy in CFS

Come back for a moment to John, and let us learn a little bit more from his experience. During our first consultation, I asked John whether he had noticed any other factors, apart from exertion, that aggravated his condition. He told me that he felt quite unwell after eating potato or wheat, but that he had not paid particular attention to this observation — he had never heard of such food reactions before. I told him that he had a classical case of CFS (in that he fulfilled all the diagnostic criteria) and that he had probably developed some degree of food intolerance as a result of his disordered immune system (which sometimes happens in CFS). I asked him to exclude all wheat and potato from his diet henceforth, and I prescribed a range of nutritional supplements. Within two weeks he felt considerably better, and within three months he wanted to get back into training! I advised against this because he had some residual symptoms, but asked him instead to embark on a graded exercise programme.

John's case illustrates a number of salient features. Firstly, he had to wait three years for an accurate diagnosis — a sad reflection on medical ignorance. Secondly, he was (as many others like him have been) sent to a psychiatrist who told him that all his symptoms were due to a depressive illness. As you will see from the discussion which follows, he was fortunate not to be accused of hysteria! Thirdly, he developed a food intolerance which significantly aggravated his symptoms. Treatment of this provided him with almost immediate improvement. Finally, he responded well to nutritional supplements. These very simple, safe and cheap measures allowed him to recover much of his lost energy, reassured him that he was not going crazy after all, and gave him a realistic hope for a full recovery. He did extremely well and now leads a normal life. Incidentally, he got that promotion!

If John had a classical case of CFS, why did his doctor not know what was wrong with him? Why did he have to wait so long for a diagnosis? Why was he told that all his symptoms were due to depression? And why did he have to wait so long for effective treatment? The answer to these questions will become clear once we have looked at the historical background to this condition.

Historical background

Contrary to popular opinion, chronic debilitating fatigue of unknown origin is not a new disease. It was first recognised as long ago as 1681 by the renowned physician Dr Thomas Sydenham. He described a chronic condition which followed hard on the heels of a fever, and which was characterised by painful and tender muscles, neurological symptoms and mood changes. He pointed out that the illness afflicted psychologically healthy individuals and, as if he could foresee the heated debate that would follow some 300 years later, he said that this illness was neither hysterical nor psychological in origin. He called the condition 'muscular rheumatism', thus emphasising two important aspects of the disease, namely, the physical nature of the illness and the muscular pain and weakness which afflicts most sufferers.

A second description appeared in 1750. In this report, Dr Manningham described the sudden onset of a chronic and debilitating illness which is indistinguishable from what we would now call CFS. He called it 'febriculae' (little fevers), thus bringing attention to the frequent low-grade temperatures that can be part of the syndrome. In 1869 the term 'neurasthenia' was introduced to emphasise the fatigue aspect of the disease (*neur*: nerves, *asthenia*: weakness).

As you can see, doctors have been grappling with unexplained fatigue for a long time, and have had great difficulty in trying to pin it down. This process has been called the framing of disease — putting an illness into a context that we can all understand and agree upon. This process is often protracted and complex, and is always subject to psychosocial pressures. For example, there is virtually no controversy nowadays in our understanding of the pathology of coronary thrombosis, but it took many years of debate and research before this state was achieved. Chronic fatigue syndrome, on the other hand, is still going through unsettling stages of heated negotiation.

The historical root of the current debate can be traced back to the closing decades of the nineteenth century, when the diagnosis of neurasthenia became very popular, especially among the well-to-do. This phenomenon was attributed to Beard, an American socialite neurologist. He was adamant that neurasthenia was largely a physical condition characterised by fatigue and other symptoms, for which he prescribed the 'rest cure'. Although this is now completely out of favour, I have included an outline of the rest cure for your interest (see insert). You will see that this could have suited many a somatiser (in that there was much to be gained by the patient). If nothing else, you will see that we have made some real progress in the past one hundred years!

Beard's original description of neurasthenia included innumerable symptoms, many of which are now known to be clearly psychiatric in origin. I have no doubt that Beard himself would agree with this if he had the benefit of our present knowledge, and we must remember the state of medical knowledge (or lack of it) that prevailed during his lifetime. For example, Dr G. V. Poore, in 1882, asserted in a medical textbook that '. . . exhaustion was characterised by loss of sleeping power, incapacity for work, inability to seriously apply the mind, headache, languor and lassitude, feeble pulse, tremor, delirium, hysteria, epilepsy, hypochondriasis, chorea, mania, and general paralysis'. We look back now aghast (with the benefit of hindsight) and marvel that all these conditions could have been thrown into one sack, but that was the way things were.

Beard's support of the physical nature of neurasthenia was challenged by a growing scepticism in medical circles, and by progress in our understanding of mental disorders. For instance, one clever chap by the name of Babinski discovered that he could distinguish between true and pseudo-epilepsy (feigned) by stroking the lateral border of the sole of the foot: the big toe goes up in the former and down in the latter. Freud also appeared on the scene at this time and described anxiety neurosis and hysteria; and then Janet described obsession and phobic disorders. Schizophrenia and melancholia (major depression) also got the attention they deserved. Finally, in 1926, Charles Dana, a professor of neurology, referred to neurasthenia as 'what we now call psychoneurosis'. As you can see, neurasthenia was an umbrella that covered a whole multitude of disparate conditions.

This evolution of psychiatric understanding and terminology rendered the diagnosis of neurasthenia almost untenable and certainly less fashionable. The popularity of neurasthenia thus declined, no doubt helped by Freud's increasing scepticism and his assertion that neurasthenia was caused by excessive masturbation. Mind you, he also said that insufficient masturbation would lead to anxiety! In spite of all this Weschler, in 1930, still felt confident enough to say: 'The suspicion is justified that true neurasthenia is an organic disease in the sense that as yet undemonstrable pathologic changes are the cause of the symptoms and not the result of psychogenic processes.' In other words, he was saying that true fatigue states of physical origin probably do exist, and that they are not 'all in the mind' — we just cannot demonstrate the underlying pathology. Nevertheless, formal interest in neurasthenia declined and was virtually lost by the 1960s, although it still appears in the current World Health Organisation International Classification of Disease (ICD-10) as defining unexplained fatigue made worse by minimal mental or physical exertion.

The rest cure (once very popular, now looked upon with disdain)

The rest cure, as described in *A Textbook of Practical Therapeutics*, 6th edn, 1897, was devised by Dr S. Weir Mitchell of Philadelphia. He was a contemporary of Beard. It was recommended 'for a large class of patients who, for various reasons, are generally ailing from apparently no organic disease, and yet whose condition is often so alarming as to lead to the belief that some hidden cause of a severe train of symptoms must be present'. This cure, it was said, 'if properly carried is often blessed with surprising results'. However, 'for the treatment to be successful the rules laid down should be rigidly followed and never remitted for a single hour'.

- Select a bright, airy, easily cleaned and comfortable room, and adjoining it, if possible, a smaller one for the nurse.
- The patient is put to bed for three to six weeks ... allowed to see no one except the nurse and the doctor, since the presence of friends requires conversation and mental effort.
- The patient, in severe cases, must be fed by the nurse ... to avoid expenditure of force required in moving the arms.
- No sitting up in bed is allowed, and if any reading is done it must be by the nurse, who can read aloud for one hour a day.

- Hair should be dressed by the nurse, to avoid effort on the part of the patient.
- To take the place of exercise . . . massage or rubbing of the body, and electricity applied to muscles.

For a typical day's existence, the physician should order the following:

7.30 a.m.	Glass of hot or cold milk.
8 a.m.	Nurse to sponge patient with tepid water, or hot and cold water alternately, to stimulate the skin and circulation, the body being wrapped in a blanket, except the portion being bathed, and dried with a rough towel to stimulate the skin.
8.30 a.m.	Breakfast: eggs, milk, or finely chopped mutton or chicken.
10 a.m.	Massage.
11 a.m.	Glass of milk, or milk-punch, or egg-nog.
12 a.m.	Reading for an hour.
1 p.m.	Dinner: small piece of steak, rare roast beef, consommé soup, mutton broth, easily digested vegetables well cooked.
3 p.m.	Electricity (to cause muscular contraction without requiring nervous energy).
4.30 p.m.	Glass of milk, or milk-punch, or egg-nog.
6.30 p.m.	Supper: very plain, no tea or coffee, toast and butter, milk, curds and whey, or a plain custard.
9.30 p.m.	Glass of milk or milk-punch.

ME and CFS

Meanwhile, several epidemics of a disease virtually indistinguishable from what we would now call CFS occurred throughout the twentieth century. The first of these occurred in 1934, in a general hospital in Los Angeles. Over 200 people, most of them doctors and nurses, were affected by a severe flu-like illness. Six months later, 55 per cent of them were still out of work. They complained, among other things, of persistent muscle pain and emotional difficulties. This outbreak was initially thought to be just another polio epidemic, but all attempts to isolate the polio virus from those affected were unsuccessful. Furthermore, it became apparent that there were definite differences between the symptoms of this illness and those of polio. The cause of the outbreak was never discovered, so they called it a 'poliomyelitis-like' illness. Many of those affected remained ill for a long time.

This epidemic was followed by others in America (1950, 1957) and in various other countries around the world. Notable among these were the outbreaks in Akureyri, Iceland (1948), the Royal Free Hospital, England (1955), and those that occurred in Australia (1949), Denmark (1953) and Switzerland (late 1930s). In fact, at least sixty recognised outbreaks have been reported to date. These have occurred among such diverse groups as military cadets, schoolteachers, school children, hospital staff, religious orders, orchestra players, research groups and, of course, whole communities. Most have been associated in some way with viral infections of various sorts: polio, Epstein-Barr, human herpes 6, coxsackie, influenza and many more besides.

Epidemics were frequently named after the location in which they occurred, thus giving rise to even more names such as Icelandic disease, Royal Free disease etc. Patients from the Royal Free epidemic were also said to have benign myalgic encephalomyelitis (ME) because they had evidence of cranial nerve palsies. Although we have inherited the ME label from that outbreak, current cases of CFS/ME are largely sporadic and show no evidence of true encephalitis (inflammation of the brain). Thus there is no evidence of the 'E' in ME.

Most modern workers therefore prefer the label 'chronic fatigue syndrome', a term coined and defined in 1988. This was the first formal recognition of the validity of chronic fatigue as a distinct clinical entity. This definition was revised in 1994 in the light of experience gained from using the first definition.

I like the term 'CFS', because it does not presume a specific pathological mechanism, but patients are still familiar with the ME label and report that the name CFS does not adequately express the distress of their illness. In America the term chronic fatigue and immune dysfunction syndrome (CFIDS) was coined in an attempt to placate this concern. However, we are not sure if the immune dysfunction is significant; and besides, not all patients have it.

Hysteria and yuppie flu

The physicians who were appointed to research the early epidemics were concerned about the lack of hard evidence of disease, and they gave due consideration to the possibility that it was just another form of hysteria. Having examined the evidence in great detail, they completely rejected this theory and stressed that it was indeed a genuine (although mysterious) illness. The fact that it could not be easily explained, or that it was hard to treat, was no reason to dismiss it as psychological in origin. This view promoted an open mind, ensured that patients were taken seriously, and encouraged continued research into the condition.

However, in 1975 two influential papers appeared in the *British Medical Journal*. The authors claimed that the Royal Free Hospital outbreak was nothing more than an outbreak of mass hysteria among impressionable nurses. As it was by now many years after the epidemic in question, the authors had no access to the patients concerned. They arrived at their conclusions by examining available medical records, and without ever setting eyes on the patients themselves. In spite of a storm of protest, and with total disregard for the findings of their eminent predecessors, these authors still managed to convince many doctors of the day that ME was a psychiatric illness. This model found favour among psychiatrists of the day and was adopted for a time. They stopped looking for an alternative explanation. Unfortunately, and to the detriment of patients, this blinkered view is still held by some today.

The media's use of terms like 'yuppie flu' is also completely erroneous in that it implies a 'new' disease of dubious origin which exclusively affects an elite group of over-ambitious and over-worked individuals. Such language only serves to stigmatise genuine patients, trivialise their illness, and isolate them even further from their families and from the sceptical doctors they look to for help.

In making the assumption of hysteria in CFS, doctors and media alike not only fail to consider the appropriate diagnostic criteria, but further fail to recognise that these people who are devastated by CFS *in no way* want to adopt the sick role for personal gain. The opposite is true. Far from bringing them gain, their illness yields nothing but the loss of reputation, social isolation and financial hardship. To them the suggestion that they are hysterical is a downright insult. The vast majority of my own patients are stable individuals who were happy with their lives until they became ill.

Case history

Sometimes the 'psychological' accusation is levelled at the person caring for the patient, rather than at the patient himself. This is what happened when 10-year-old Carl became ill. He was a happy child who came from a secure and loving family. He was very popular in his local school, where he excelled. He enjoyed all sports, but was particularly addicted to football, and he used to have long chats with his dad about every player in the professional league.

He then developed a sore throat, followed by headache, bellyache and sore muscles. He became so weak he had to be admitted to hospital, where every possible investigation was carried out. As is often the case in this condition, all the results were normal. At visiting time, his mother used to help him walk up and down the hospital corridor — his own legs being too weak to carry him. The consultant in charge of his case saw what was happening and reprimanded the mother for not letting the lad stand on his own two feet. 'Let him go', he said. So she let him go and he fell to the ground. With tears in her eyes, and bewilderment in the lad's, she picked him up again. After some more harsh words from the doctor, Carl's mother was left in no doubt that she was being held responsible for the child's plight. The consultant told her that she was an 'over-involved mother', and that Carl would get better as soon as she stopped fussing over him.

Of course she was anxious and upset — she had every reason to be! She was a good mother who had watched her happy-go-lucky and energetic son decline into immobility, pain and frustration. He was young, with his whole life before him, and he had been devastated by a mysterious illness which the doctor could not explain, except on the basis of her inadequacy as a parent; nor could he offer any treatment apart from harsh and inexcusable words whose only effect was to add insult to injury. Carl and his mother felt hurt and let down by the uncaring and dismissive attitude of the medical profession. Having been thus deprived of proper advice and support, they felt isolated and confused.

He was discharged from hospital, having been told that he would get better within three weeks, but when I first saw him some five months later, he was no better. He complained of persistent muscle pain and weakness. He was still not able to walk, and he complained of daily headache, bellyache and 'sore sinuses'.

His mother brought him to the door in a wheelchair. He then slid on to the floor in the hall and hobbled the short distance to my consulting room on his *knees*. This he was able to do, but he could not walk on his feet. He was also able to move his arms fairly well, and these he used to great advantage in playing ball with his mates, and pushing himself along on his skateboard (he used to sit on the board and push off the ground with his hands). However, this activity left him feeling exhausted for the next few days.

What I found particularly interesting about Carl was how he had — without anatomical knowledge — perfectly identified his most severely affected muscles. These were the quadriceps (front thigh), hamstrings (back thigh) and gastrocnemius (calf) muscles. All these were tender to touch and painful when stretched. These muscles move the knee and ankle joints, and without them normal walking is impossible. Carl would not have known that he should still be able to 'walk' on his knees, even when all his leg muscles were sore and weak. To walk on his knees, he only needs to move his hip joint, and this he can do by calling on an entirely separate group of muscles from those already mentioned, the ilio-psoas (which is inside the abdomen) and the gluteal muscles (the buttock). Whilst relying on these muscles to hobble around, he is able to rest his most severely affected muscle groups. Hysterical people are not so clever at anatomy!

Carl did not respond to treatment as John did. There were other treatment options available, but these were still experimental (in that their worth had not yet been established by clinical trials) and he had not yet decided what to do about them. He needed to be wary of the numerous quacks who

233

offered him false hope with magical cures, and who were likely to demand considerable financial rewards for their wizardry.

Carl needed close supervision over the following months. We had to watch out for the social and psychological pressures which any chronic and debilitating disease would bring into a young life. We gave him as much symptomatic relief as possible, as much information about the illness as we had, consistent support and, above all, time. We told him it would be hard, but that time would eventually heal in the vast majority of cases. He mourned the loss of his independence, the loss of his peer group, and the loss of all that he enjoyed doing with his energy.

His friends were terrific at first, but then they stopped calling. Were they getting fed up? Did they find it too painful to watch, or did they feel too awkward in his presence? He could have developed a bitter resentment against those who tried to care for him. He could also have become depressed and, if he did, would not that be an understandable reaction?

Carl remained ill for the best part of two years. For much of that time he was chair-bound. There was, therefore, a degree of urgency about the case. He had spent so long in a wheelchair that we were afraid he would be permanently disabled if we failed to mobilise him now. He finally agreed to see another paediatrician, a kind and considerate man. You can imagine Carl's reluctance to go back into hospital after his previous experience, but he went in anyway. He was desperate. Whilst there, he had intensive (albeit graded) physiotherapy. I am happy to report that he has never looked back. He now plays football regularly with one of the local clubs and leads a virtually normal life.

Lessons from history

History is littered with sad reminders of man's inability to live side by side with what he cannot control or understand. Doctors are no exception to this. In times past, they told patients they were ill because they had sinned; treated headache by drilling holes in the skull; 'cured' constipation by removing the large bowel; dealt with (female) hysteria by excising genitalia; offered to sterilise epileptics for eugenic reasons, and locked the insane in deplorable dungeons. We look back now incredulous at such barbaric treatment, but what about us? Have present day doctors 'arrived'? Have we learned all we need to learn? Or can we, with humility, learn from each other and from our patients — as the patriarchs did from theirs?

Take the bubonic plague, for instance. It swept across Europe in the fourteenth century, leaving millions dead in its wake. It was a mysterious disease in that nobody knew the cause or the cure. It was merciless and no respecter of persons. The young and the old, the rich and the poor, the mad and the not-so-mad, were all fair game. No one knew who its next victim would be. Explanations were desperately sought and doctors came under great pressure to provide the answers. Some said it was caused by 'invisible particles in the air', others suspected 'poisoned wells' or 'bouts of riotous living', and Nero's bigoted descendants blamed the Jews. Psychiatrists, unfortunately, had not yet been invented, so we don't know what explanations they might have offered!

News of a fresh wave of death in a nearby village brought terror to the hearts of a defenceless people. How could you fight an enemy you could not see? They fearfully locked themselves away, barring the door against all intruders, preferring to live reclusive lives rather than face the Black Death. Those who could afford it would abandon their village homes and move deep into the countryside, remaining there until the coast was clear again at home. The doctors were just as frustrated as everybody else. In their search for an effective cure, they made all sorts of recommendations to their patients: 'burn aromatic woods and herbs'; 'try sleeping in a different position' or 'eat a special diet.' Braver patients, who obviously had great trust in their doctors, allowed themselves to be repeatedly bled. Such treatment was quite common in those days, and is still used today in certain circumstances. Richer patients were subjected to a different sort of bleeding: they were offered very expensive medical cocktails of gold and pearls (gold is still used therapeutically today, but not for the bubonic plague)!

It was said in those days that 'every expert held his own opinion and offered his own cure'. But the truth of the matter is that they were no more effective than their white-robed 'flagellant brethren', who went from village to village with the sign of the cross, whipping themselves in the forlorn hope of appeasing an angry God. It would be centuries before the condition was fully understood: the plague is caused by *Yersinia pestis*, a microorganism which normally infects rats. Rodent fleas, which feed on dying rats, spread the infection to other rats and infect humans as well — in much the same way as the mosquito transmits malaria. Once humans were infected with the germ, they passed it on to others in saliva droplets. Effective preventative measures are based on a clear understanding of the causative agent, and lifesaving treatment is directed at eradicating the offending germ from the body.

Of course, we do not need to go back that far in history to find other examples of error. Patients who became ill with Lyme disease, for instance, were told that their illness was psychiatric in nature — until the discovery in the 1980s of the offending bug (pages 195). Similarly, patients from the Pacific rim were told that their mysterious symptoms were psychological in nature — until the discovery of ciguatoxin, a nerve poison found in contaminated fish. We are still vulnerable to error.

CFS is a mysterious illness. We do not yet know what causes it, or how to cure it. Every expert holds his own opinion, and offers his own cure. Patients caught in the middle are understandably confused. Those who have been summarily dismissed by the medical profession will turn to non-medical practitioners. Here, if they are lucky, they will meet the first person who was ever willing to give them time, and listen to their story sympathetically. They may even be given appropriate advice with regard to rest, activity, diet and nutritional supplements. If they are less fortunate, they will find themselves at the mercy of unscrupulous mercenaries, and be subjected to all sorts of expensive and questionable treatments.

From Controversy to
23 Consensus in CFS

Many patients with CFS develop neuropsychiatric symptoms during the course of their illness. The most common of these are cognitive impairment (poor memory and concentration), anxiety and depression. At least half of all patients can expect to be affected by these at some stage and to some degree during their illness. Research suggests that the anxiety and depression of CFS are best understood as a reaction to the illness, rather than the cause of it; and that the cognitive impairment cannot be explained merely by anxiety and/or depression. In other words, cognitive impairment is an inherent part of the illness (hence its inclusion in the diagnostic criteria), whereas depression/anxiety, if they are present, are the result of the illness. Furthermore, the severity of psychiatric symptoms is directly related to the severity of the fatigue. Surely this is exactly what we would expect. The longer we are ill, and the more ill we are, the more likely we are to become depressed or anxious about our illness. So, then, we readily admit that psychiatric symptoms overlap with CFS in many cases, but we contend that this is entirely understandable.

However, the overlap of psychiatric symptoms with CFS does not sit comfortably with the medical profession, and has given rise to several schools of opposing thought. Some say that CFS is merely a socio-cultural phenomenon (a fashionable disease); others say it's a psychodynamic dysfunction (e.g. suppressed rage); some believe it's a psychiatric disorder (e.g. hysteria); and some believe it's a physical illness. Finally, some doctors assert that CFS does not even exist. You may have met one of these. If so, you will recognise this short scene. 'Doctor, do you think I might have ME?' The doctor replies, with an angry and dismissive wave of the hand, 'ME? There's no such thing.'

Depression in CFS

Let us take a closer look at depression in the context of chronic fatigue syndrome. Why do some patients become depressed during their CFS and others do not? There are three factors to consider. Firstly, the original infecting virus may penetrate the brain cells of some patients. In doing so, the cells are not destroyed (which would be catastrophic), but their function may be severely disrupted. This alone could give rise to psychiatric symptoms, such as mood changes, irritability, difficulty with memory and concentration, headache, sleep disturbance and fatigue etc. Secondly, the pain and debility which are part and parcel of the disease, and the inevitable loss of independence and dignity which ensue, are not easy to put up with. These all add to the total load of stress on the individual patient, and stress (as we have seen in Chapter 4) may lead to depression, particularly in those who are genetically vulnerable.

Thirdly, patients with CFS are often greeted with suspicion by their doctors. And as we have seen, they may be accused of hysteria (or malingering for that matter). These destructive attitudes amount to a condescending value judgment, and they are difficult to bear. They isolate patients from their doctors, as well as from their families and friends. 'After all', these will say, 'if the doctor says there's nothing wrong with you, then it must be true.' Employers also become impatient at the amount of sick leave that has been taken, particularly in the absence of a doctor's certificate, and the threat of dismissal is raised. The hapless patient tries harder, but the physical and mental effort involved only serve to worsen his condition. Now, ask yourself honestly: would you get depressed in this situation? I know I would.

So why don't all doctors see it like this? And what reasons do the sceptics give for their stance? We must try to be fair here, and give a little ground. We must acknowledge that:

- Fatigue may be the covert forerunner of depression.
- The symptoms of CFS are commonly seen in depressive and anxiety states.
- Depression may be disguised by the subtlety of a smile, or the complexity of hypochondriasis.
- Depressive illness may be precipitated by physical stress such

as a surgical operation *or an infection*.
- We have not yet developed a reliable diagnostic test for CFS, hence we cannot 'prove' that it exists.

These are reasonable arguments, and they explain why some very good doctors are reluctant to accept that CFS is a valid diagnosis. Having said that, we should counter with the sobering reminder that the most common mistake in medicine is the assumption of psychological illness in the absence of physical signs of disease; and that psychiatric features, if present, may be caused by physical disease.

In any case, there is a growing body of clinical and research evidence which supports the view that CFS is, in fact, a distinct clinical entity. In the first place, there are crucial differences between what doctors call major (clinical) depression and CFS, although these differences may be lost when the former complicates the latter. Briefly stated, patients with major depression usually feel utterly dejected. They find themselves overwhelmed by feelings of guilt, failure and low self-esteem. They may feel that they are being punished for previous misdemeanours, and they often contemplate suicide. They have no interest in life; nor can they find pleasure in any pursuit. Sex, food, hobbies, good books and films all lose their appeal. Physical exercise and, interestingly, short-term sleep deprivation may alleviate some of their symptoms for a while.

CFS patients, on the other hand, seldom feel guilty. They have a good self-image, although this may become eroded as time goes by. They feel a sense of pressure to recover ('Are you *still* tired all the time?') but they do not have a sense of failure. They maintain an active interest in life that is frustrated only by the limitations imposed on them by the illness, and they still find pleasure in sex, food, books, films and their more sedate hobbies. Their mood may well be low, but is seldom one of utter dejection. Consequently, suicide is rare — but remains a risk for those most severely affected. Finally, and this is a very important point, physical exertion and sleep deprivation are guaranteed to worsen their symptoms — so much so, that if they do feel better after exercise, the diagnosis of CFS is untenable.

These distinctions are perhaps most clearly seen when the same patient suffers from CFS and major depression at different stages in his/her life. The patient is able to see the clear and unmistakable contrast that exists between the two states.

Case history

James is a case in point. He had a severe viral infection when he was 16 years old which put him to bed for two weeks. He remained chronically fatigued and had all the symptoms of CFS for the next eighteen months. He had the good sense to rest completely in the initial stages of his illness. He stayed away from school for a while, and never attempted to play rugby, his favourite pastime. Nor did he engage in any other activity that would have left him feeling tired.

Towards the end of his eighteen month illness, he started to feel well, and shortly after that he was back to his normal self. He held a full-time summer job, walked a few miles each day between home and workplace, and started training with the rugby team on alternate days. By the end of that summer he was free of all symptoms (yes, people *do* recover from CFS with time).

Then he had the misfortune of a broken romance, and we all know how painful that can be. His thoughts became filled with a sense of loss, and the world around him lost its appeal. Within weeks he was questioning the meaning of life, the whereabouts of God, and 'Who was I anyway?' He remembers one night in particular, as he stood gazing at a starry sky, being struck with the enormity of the universe and feeling that he was just a drop in the ocean, an insignificant and transient dweller on the face of an enormous planet. Death was on his mind. He could see no purpose in living and he thought about throwing himself into the river. He had lost the will to fight. He felt exhausted, his concentration was poor, he was not sleeping well, and he vomited most of the little food he ate. His parents, alarmed at the rapid deterioration in his condition, wondered whether he had entered a relapse of his CFS, but John could tell the difference. It was not CFS, it was depression — and he knew it. This sort of profound questioning is not unusual in teenage years. It has to do with forming a sense of identity and purpose.

It is interesting to note that formal psychological tests, such as the Minnesota Multiphasic Personality Inventory (MMPI), also distinguish CFS from mental illnesses. The MMPI, which is used by psychiatrists in over ninety countries, provides valuable help in discerning between depression, hysteria and hypochondriasis. Patients with CFS who have been assessed by the MMPI do not fit into any of these recognised categories: they have a unique profile — a signature pattern, as it were — which adds weight to the argument that CFS is a distinct clinical entity with its own features. Furthermore, and contrary to popular opinion, systematic assessments of personality in CFS reveal that personality type has nothing to do with the illness. Thus, perfectionist and obsessive personalities are no more or less likely to succumb than anyone else.

In all of this we must not forget that many patients with CFS do not become depressed or unduly anxious. These are the fortunate ones who have been blessed twice: the first time round, with a robust mental health, and the second, with a brain which has escaped the worst ravages of viral infiltration.

Case history

Mary is one such girl. She had enjoyed sixteen years of near perfect health and was doing well at school, until the summer of 1989 when she came down with glandular fever. She had the classical sore throat, the swollen glands and a positive blood test. She simply never recovered her full strength, nor anything like it, and she was unable to return to school for one full year. After that year, she started to study again and coped quite well (as long as she had ten hours' sleep at night — an increase on her previous sleep requirement). In spite of her continued headaches, muscle pains and exhaustion, Mary would have told you that she was 'all right' during those days. She is not the complaining sort.

She managed to carry on like this until the winter of 92. She then caught another cold which knocked her back considerably. The pain in her back and legs and the headaches became more severe. She felt dizzy and nauseated, and she was utterly, I mean utterly, exhausted. She also admitted to many other symptoms: palpitations, drenching sweats, joint pains, bloating of the abdomen and bouts of diarrhoea. Her concentration and memory were abysmal. This relapse could not have come at a worse time, in that she was, by now, in her final year at school, and her performance in the forthcoming exams would determine her future career. I first saw her at this time, when she was three years into her illness.

Having already lost out on one year, she did not relish the prospect of losing another, especially after preparing so hard for her exams. She hoped to recover some mental energy so that she could at least sit the exams as planned. To this end, Mary embarked on a dietary investigation for associated food intolerance. She felt a small but significant improvement in her mental ability within two weeks, and another small improvement over the following month. Nutritional supplements were also prescribed at that time. She felt well enough to sit the exams, although she needed one-to-one supervision in a separate classroom. This allowed her to push her paper to one side every now and again and lay her head on the desk for a rest. She collapsed in a heap after this enormous mental and physical effort. Needless to say, she felt that she had not done herself justice at all; but when the results were made available, she discovered that she had done exceptionally well and had secured her first choice of both faculty and university. Throughout all this time, she never once became depressed. Yes, she was frustrated, and yes, she was (and still is) impatient for recovery, but her mood has remained noticeably stable.

As she is now too exhausted to entertain thoughts of further study, the university has kindly kept her place open for the start of the next academic year, by which time we all hope she will have recovered. She is currently on a course of treatment with this goal in mind.

The contribution of research

The past decade has seen a significant growth in CFS research. This work has generated over 700 articles on the subject and is changing our perception of the illness. To my mind, the most exciting findings are those which hint at possible pathological mechanisms. If we could unravel these, we could then work on a reliable diagnostic test, further establish the validity of CFS, and explore new avenues of treatment.

At this point, and without wishing to get lost in scientific detail, I would like to highlight some of the key research findings that have been reported to date, particularly in relation to depression. We can now say with some degree of scientific confidence that CFS and depression are not the same illness. You may recall that depression has a biological substrate — a physical mode of expression (page 32). Although we cannot be sure of the precise mechanisms involved, we can see evidence of disturbed brain and hormone function in depression, especially in the hypothalamic-pituitary-adrenal (HPA) axis. A properly functioning HPA axis is crucial to health. It helps to regulate biological rhythms (including the sleep/wake cycle), appetite, mood, immune function, temperature regulation and hormones. It is readily apparent that any disturbance of the HPA axis could lead to many symptoms. Notable among these are marked fatigue, sleep disorders, food cravings, altered mood and abnormal sweating.

Specifically, we know that depression is associated with:

- an increase in cortisol production generally (the adrenal gland responding to messages from the brain).
- an increase in brain cortisol.
- a reduced sensitivity in the hypothalamus to cortisol.
- reduced serotonin neurotransmission in the brain.

We can also measure these same parameters in CFS, and compare them to depression. What we find is that in CFS:

- There is a decrease in cortisol production generally.
- There is a decrease in brain cortisol.
- There is an increased sensitivity in the hypothalamus.
- There is an increase of serotonin activity in the brain (although this activity is defective).

Thus, not only are depression and CFS seen to be different; they are in some respects polar opposites! Depression is associated with hyperactivation of the HPA axis and hypercortisolaemia, whereas CFS is associated with hypoactivation and hypocortisolaemia.

You are probably aware of the fact that cortisol is one of the main steroid hormones in the body, and that we can administer cortisone as a medicine. You may wonder then what would happen if we gave cortisone to CFS patients. Would it help? In fact, it does; but only a little, and the side effects are unacceptable. This finding (low cortisol which does not respond well to supplemental cortisol) suggests that the brain is not responding well to steroid messages.

In fact, we now have evidence to suggest that several pathways in the brain are disrupted in some way in CFS patients. But please do not be frightened by this. The disruption is functional. The brain cells themselves would look normal to the naked eye, or on a scan. They are just not working properly.

Many other aspects of CFS have been studied, and some of these are potentially important. I would like to draw your attention to just one more interesting area, because I think we will hear more about this in the years ahead. A defect has been found in the 2-5 oligoadenylate synthetase/RNase antiviral pathway (sorry about the name!), and this may be corrected with a modified RNA drug (Ampligen). Early clinical trials suggest that this could be an effective treatment for patients with CFS who are failing to progress with other forms of treatment.

Now that is interesting, isn't it? We have just seen two completely different areas of research into the same condition, both of which show promise. How can this be? It is my belief, and this is shared by many colleagues, that what we now call CFS is in fact a collection of different conditions which share a final common pathway. I can foresee, one hundred years from now, that some youngster will write a book about this, in which he/she will marvel at our blindness in much the same way that we marvel at that of our predecessors. Neurasthenia was a very large umbrella that covered many diverse conditions, and I believe that CFS will turn out to be just as broad a covering.

Towards consensus

The first real step towards consensus was taken in 1988, when the Centre for Disease Control (CDC) in the USA offered its first definition of chronic fatigue syndrome. This was the first formal recognition of the illness. In 1991, the Oxford group offered its definition and suggested guidelines for research. Then in 1994 the CDC revised its definition in the hope of providing a more suitable instrument for clinical and research purposes. The next step towards consensus came in October 1996, when a joint working party from the Royal Colleges of Physicians, Psychiatrists and General Practitioners, at the request of the Chief Medical Officer, published a report on chronic fatigue syndrome, and an updated version in 1997. The authors of this report had extensive clinical experience of chronic unexplained fatigue. In summary, they concluded that:

- CFS is the preferred term for the disorder.
- The aetiology (cause) of CFS is little understood, although there is some evidence that specific viral agents (glandular fever, meningitis etc.) may trigger CFS.
- The likelihood of CFS is increased where there is evidence of excessive fatigue and/or psychological morbidity before acquiring an infection.
- CFS is widespread, with a prevalence in the region of 0.5%.
- The majority of patients with CFS have co-morbid psychological conditions. Over half those presenting with CFS have mood disorders and a further quarter show evidence of anxiety or somatisation disorders.
- The suggestion of a social class relationship (implicit in the term 'yuppie flu') should be dismissed as due to bias.
- CFS occurs in children, and though most can be managed in primary care with the involvement of school nurses and school authorities, some will need referral to specialist units.
- CFS is making substantial demands on primary and secondary care health services.
- The total social and economic costs associated with the functional impairment of CFS are considerable.

The report also lays stress on:

- The benefits of early treatment in primary care with a view to preventing chronic disability.
- The importance of striking a balance between over and under investigation.

- The importance of the doctor accepting that the patient's distress is genuine.
- The importance of being prepared to treat the patient.
- The detrimental effects of bed rest.
- The potential benefits of controlled increases in activity, including graded exercise.
- The potential benefits of cognitive behavioural therapy.
- The need to treat concurrent psychiatric disorders.
- The need for trials to evaluate the role of antidepressants as an adjunct to treatment even when no depression is present.

I also like the report's advice to sceptical doctors. I quote:'There is no place in the clinical consultation for such statements as "There is nothing wrong with you", or "It is all in the mind", just as there is no place for such statements as "You have ME — there is nothing I can do." A doctor may have doubts about the nosological status (validity) of CFS, but it is unacceptable and counterproductive to add this scepticism to the distress of chronically fatigued patients.'

By and large, this report was well received and seen as a significant contribution towards consensus. However, objections have been voiced to a perceived over-representation of psychiatric models, and to the blanket recommendation for graded exercise which is considered by some to be not appropriate for all patients. More of this anon.

Assessing the Impact
24 of Chronic Fatigue

By definition, patients with CFS will suffer significantly in terms of their health-related quality of life and work. As we have seen, the diagnostic criteria for the disorder require a substantial reduction in previous levels of functional activity, but what does that really mean? Let us take a closer look at the specifics of functional impairment.

Formal studies into this aspect of CFS have been few and far between, but those that have appeared suggest that affected patients do indeed suffer profound losses in all major domains of life, including physical, psychological and social functioning. Furthermore, the severe personal and financial burdens of this illness have implications beyond the individual patient. Their families and friends suffer with them empathetically, as well as having their own unique frustrations and burdens to bear. Partners may find themselves with added responsibilities for finance, housework and child rearing. Similarly, workmates may try to cover for the patient, but this becomes increasingly difficult as time goes by. Employers come under pressure to replace them, and their careers are put on hold. Many find it impossible to hold a meaningful personal conversation, let alone socialise in a crowd. Some complain of great difficulty in trying to maintain their hobbies, and most find it almost impossible to conduct their academic pursuits with the vigour they would like. As for sport, forget it! Meanwhile, the patient may be reduced from a 'contributing' member of the economy to a 'receiving' one, in need of social welfare support. The demands placed on the health services are also considerable, both in terms of time and expense.

There are several instruments used in research for assessing specific quality of life issues. The parameters examined include:

- the ability to function physically and socially
- the severity of pain (if present)
- general feelings of health and vitality (or lack thereof)
- mental health, and
- emotional functioning.

CFS patients have significantly low scores in all but one of these parameters. Admittedly, there is great variability between individuals, but this comes as no great surprise. There is a spectrum of illness, from mild to severe, with many grades of impairment in between. It is also quite possible for patients to fluctuate during the course of their illness, sometimes feeling better and other times worse.

The exception to the rule is interesting. CFS patients, in the throes of their illness, produce normal scores in the emotional domain. This suggests that although quality of life is profoundly impaired, patients with CFS do not allow their emotions to interfere with their daily roles or activities. In other words, it is not just a question of them saying 'I don't feel like doing it' — they can't do it!

What about your fatigue?

Perhaps you have never thought about the particular impact that fatigue has had on your life. In that case, what you are working on is a general impression of illness and debility, rather than an exact measure. If so, I would suggest that you take time out to identify some specifics.

Have a look at the following questionnaire. It is not offered as a scientific instrument but as a simple clinical aid. You may feel that some of the questions are irrelevant, but consider them anyway. They do need to be asked, and answered. I trust that their relevance will become clear later on. This exercise will help you to clarify your present state in terms of your functional ability, your most troublesome symptoms, the losses you have suffered and the pressures you are currently under. It will also make you think about the possible contributing factors that led to your illness in the first place; and finally, it will provide you with a baseline from which you can construct a management plan for recovery.

Fatigue impact assessment

GENERAL

1. How long have you been fatigued?
   - ❏ less than 1 year
   - ❏ 1–2 years
   - ❏ 2–4 years
   - ❏ 5–10 years
   - ❏ more than 10 years

2. When did your fatigue start? Exact date if known:

3. Did your fatigue start
   - ❏ suddenly
   - ❏ gradually
   - ❏ intermittently

4. Did you experience a flu-like illness prior to the onset of your fatigue?
   - ❏ yes   ❏ no

5. What do you think is the cause of your fatigue?

6. Would you say that your fatigue is
   - ❏ mostly physical
   - ❏ mostly psychological
   - ❏ a bit of both

7. Compared to previous levels, what is your current level of activity
   - ❏ 0–20%
   - ❏ 21–40%
   - ❏ 41–60%
   - ❏ 61–80%
   - ❏ 81–100%

8. In general, would say you are
   - ❏ getting better
   - ❏ getting worse
   - ❏ staying the same

9. Did you experience stressful life events prior to the onset of your illness?

PSYCHOSOCIAL ASPECTS

10. Throughout your illness, have you found your family
    - ☐ very supportive
    - ☐ supportive
    - ☐ not so supportive
    - ☐ not at all supportive

11. Throughout your illness, have you found your friends
    - ☐ very supportive
    - ☐ supportive
    - ☐ not so supportive
    - ☐ not at all supportive

12. Throughout your illness, have you found doctors
    - ☐ very supportive
    - ☐ supportive
    - ☐ not so supportive
    - ☐ not at all supportive

13. Have you lost friendships as a result of this illness? ☐ yes ☐ no

14. Have you suffered stressful life events during this illness? ☐ yes ☐ no

15. Have you suffered financially as a result of this illness? ☐ yes ☐ no

SLEEP QUALITY AND PATTERN

During the past month, would you say that

16. My sleep is as refreshing as it used to be ☐ yes ☐ no

17. My sleep pattern is disturbed ☐ yes ☐ no

18. I sleep more than I did before I became ill ☐ yes ☐ no

19. I sleep less than I did before I became ill ☐ yes ☐ no

20. I have difficulty getting to sleep ☐ yes ☐ no

21. I have difficulty staying asleep ☐ yes ☐ no

22. I have difficulty waking up ☐ yes ☐ no

23. I take a daytime sleep ❑ yes ❑ no

24. How many hours' sleep do you get every day?
❑ less than 4 hrs
❑ 4–6 hrs
❑ 7–8 hrs
❑ 9–10 hrs
❑ more than 10 hrs

OCCUPATIONAL/ACADEMIC ASPECTS

Tick the statement which best describes your condition:

25. I am totally unable to work/study ❑ yes ❑ no

26. I am able for part-time work/study, but suffer a restricted social life ❑ yes ❑ no

27. I am able for part-time work/study, and enjoy a good social life ❑ yes ❑ no

28. I am able for full-time work/study, but suffer a restricted social life ❑ yes ❑ no

29. I am able for full-time work/study, and enjoy a good social life ❑ yes ❑ no

PERSONAL AND DOMESTIC ASPECTS

During the past month

30. I have been more or less bed-bound ❑ yes ❑ no

31. I stay out of bed during my waking hours ❑ yes ❑ no ❑ with difficulty

32. I go back to bed during my waking hours ❑ yes ❑ no ❑ sometimes

33. I need help with all aspects of personal care ❑ yes ❑ no

34. I am able to dress myself ❑ yes ❑ no ❑ with difficulty

35. I am able to wash myself ❑ yes ❑ no ❑ with difficulty

251

36. I am able to wash my hair   ❐ yes   ❐ no
    ❐ with difficulty

37. I am able to dry my hair   ❐ yes   ❐ no
    ❐ with difficulty

38. I am able to prepare meals   ❐ yes   ❐ no
    ❐ with difficulty

39. I am able to feed myself   ❐ yes   ❐ no
    ❐ with difficulty

40. I am able to do light housework
(e.g. make a bed, wash the dishes)   ❐ yes   ❐ no
    ❐ with difficulty

41. I am able to do heavy housework
(e.g. iron clothes, wash a floor)   ❐ yes   ❐ no
    ❐ with difficulty

42. I am able to receive visitors   ❐ yes   ❐ no
    ❐ with difficulty

43. I am able to accept phone calls   ❐ yes   ❐ no
    ❐ with difficulty

44. I am house-bound   ❐ no   ❐ yes

45. I am able to go out of the house   ❐ yes   ❐ no
    ❐ with difficulty

46. I am able to shop for basic necessities   ❐ yes   ❐ no
    ❐ with difficulty

47. I am able to shop for other items   ❐ yes   ❐ no
    ❐ with difficulty

48. I am able to care for others ❐ n/a
(e.g. children, spouse, parent etc.)   ❐ yes   ❐ no
    ❐ with difficulty

49. I can engage in meaningful
conversation   ❐ yes   ❐ no
    ❐ with difficulty

50. I can read for pleasure   ❐ yes   ❐ no
    ❐ with difficulty

51. I can write   ❐ yes   ❐ no
    ❐ with difficulty

52. I can watch television   ❐ yes   ❐ no
    ❐ with difficulty

53. I am able to engage in sexual activity   ❐ n/a   ❐ yes   ❐ no   ❐ with difficulty

54. I am able to engage in light exercise   ❐ yes   ❐ no
     (e.g. gentle walking)   ❐ with difficulty

55. I am able to engage in vigorous   ❐ yes   ❐ no
     exercise (e.g. cycling, jogging)   ❐ with difficulty

56. I am able to engage in sport   ❐ yes   ❐ no
                                ❐ with difficulty

ASSOCIATED SYMPTOMS

During the past month, and while you are at rest, have you experienced

57. Muscle pain	❐ none	❐ some	❐ a lot
58. Joint pain	❐ none	❐ some	❐ a lot
59. Headache	❐ none	❐ some	❐ a lot
60. Difficulties with memory	❐ none	❐ some	❐ a lot
61. Difficulties with concentration	❐ none	❐ some	❐ a lot
62. Sore throats	❐ none	❐ some	❐ a lot
63. Sore glands	❐ none	❐ some	❐ a lot
64. Low mood	❐ none	❐ some	❐ a lot
65. Anxiety	❐ none	❐ some	❐ a lot

Others: specify

66.	❐ some	❐ a lot
67.	❐ some	❐ a lot
68.	❐ some	❐ a lot

The full spectrum of functional impairment

Patients often ask me to quantify their fatigue: 'How bad am I, doctor?' But the truth of the matter is that we cannot quantify fatigue other than in terms of the impact it has on your activity. At one end of the scale, we find some patients who are bedridden and in need of constant help and personal care. They have to be washed, dressed, spoon-fed and carried to the bathroom. At the other end of the scale, we find people who are well on the road to recovery and complain only of minimal symptoms. Some of these manage to function fairly well, but others are still paying a price. The latter can maintain their essential functions, such as home-making or bread-winning, but they expend every ounce of energy in doing so, and have nothing left to give at the end of the day. Some patients will tell us that they can do almost everything that is required of them, but it takes all their effort.

Various scales have been devised in an attempt to grade the severity of fatigue, but these are still subjective measures of how you feel yourself. So the only person who can really answer the question of functional ability is you. This is more complex than may first appear, because it raises questions of motivation, caution, frustration, fear (of making things worse) and so on. I am also frequently asked in this context whether a patient should be doing more, or less, as the case may be. These issues will be addressed in the next chapter.

25 The Treatment of Chronic Fatigue

The treatment and care of many chronic disorders is, *ipso facto*, unsatisfactory. This is as true for chronic fatigue as for any other illness. Indeed, chronic fatigue syndrome (CFS) has assumed a formidable reputation for being difficult to treat. This is not helped by the controversy which has dogged the condition through the years, nor by the fact that the medical profession does not yet have an evidence-based consensus protocol of care. In other words, doctors do not yet agree on how the condition should be treated. This means that patients presenting with chronic debilitating fatigue do so to a divided profession. It is reasonable to assume then that the quality of medical care you receive will depend, at least in part, on the attitudes, knowledge and beliefs of the individual doctors you happen to consult. Family doctors, for their part, are not happy with this state of affairs and express dissatisfaction with the quality of care fatigued patients receive, both from themselves as primary care physicians and from their referrals to specialist centres.

Most of the published research on the treatment and outcome of CFS has come from specialist centres. The overall impression they give us is one of a dismal outlook. However, there is ample evidence to suggest that many doctors do not refer their fatigued patients for a second opinion. This means that specialist centres are not seeing the full spectrum of illness, and it is quite likely that they only get to see the worst-affected cases. There is little doubt in my mind that this explains the poor prognosis reported by these centres, and that these reports, in turn, have contributed to the culture of 'treatment nihilism' within the medical profession.

In my experience, the vast majority of CFS patients regain a substantial degree of functional activity and a decent quality of life. We can even go further than that and declare that a significant number get to a stage where they consider themselves fully recovered. We need to rid ourselves of the notion that nothing can be done for the fatigued. It simply isn't true.

You should aim for full functional recovery in all domains of life, although I admit that in practice this may require changes in lifestyle or personal ambition, particularly if these are unreasonable. There are several principles of management that can help you achieve this, and these can be adopted by all patients with fatigue, whatever its severity.

Principles of management: 1. Get a diagnosis

I know it seems a rather obvious thing to say, but your first task is to get a diagnosis for your fatigue. This will be of benefit to you, your family, your friends, your employer and your doctor. A diagnosis . . .

- helps to consolidate the therapeutic relationship that exists between you and your doctor.
- prevents unnecessary investigations.
- reduces anxiety (at least I know what I have).
- reduces expense.
- allows you to name your distress.
- helps you come to terms with your illness.
- prevents potentially harmful 'doctor-shopping'.
- protects you from further disability.
- gives a structure for understanding your predicament.
- provides a framework for a sensible and pragmatic plan of action.
- helps to enlist the support of family, friends and employers.

What should my doctor do?

The doctor will need to fully evaluate your fatigue before offering a diagnosis. This may take some time. As always in medicine, this process includes a thorough clinical history, followed by a physical examination and appropriate laboratory tests. It should be possible to get to a working diagnosis, even if it is the less satisfactory label of 'idiopathic fatigue'. At the very least, other explanations of fatigue can be ruled out. It may be helpful for you to see the sort of questions and tests you can expect from your doctor when you present with a chief complaint of chronic debilitating fatigue.

CLINICAL HISTORY

Your doctor will enquire about:

1. Mode of onset — was it gradual or sudden? Many patients will pinpoint the onset to a specific date, and this may suggest a precipitating event(s). Your doctor knows, however, that such recall is subject to rationalisation — a retrospective tendency we all engage in, in an attempt to understand our present distress. You may be asked to express your beliefs and attributions. For example, some patients attribute their fatigue to a specific viral illness, such as glandular fever, and will volunteer that they have not felt well since they contracted it; others may identify one or more adverse life events, such as marital break-down, a road traffic accident, or bereavement. Twenty per cent of patients will say that their fatigue was of very gradual onset, becoming worse over months or years. In these cases you may be asked:'When did you last feel perfectly well?' 'What was the first indication that something was amiss?', or 'When did you first go to a doctor seeking help for your fatigue?' With these questions, your doctor is looking for some indication as to the duration of your fatigue and its possible underlying cause(s).

2. Psychosocial influences prior to or concurrent with fatigue onset, and specifically about prolonged stressful situations (work, relationships etc.) which are known to adversely affect sleep quality, immune function and mood. However, social adversity is by no means always associated with fatigue onset (or delayed recovery).

3. Mood changes, cognitive difficulty and alterations in personality, with particular attention to current depression and/or anxiety, self-destructive thoughts and psychomotor retardation.

4. The current use of drugs, including prescribed medicines as well as over-the-counter preparations and alcohol and substance abuse. All these drugs can cause fatigue and depression in susceptible people.

5. Sleep quality and patterns, looking for evidence of a sleep disorder. You will be asked to distinguish between the feelings of 'fatigue' and 'excessive daytime sleepiness'.
6. Associated symptoms, especially criterion B symptoms (listed on page 221).
7. Functional impairment — what is the precise impact of your fatigue?

PHYSICAL EXAMINATION

After the history, you will be offered a physical examination. There are no specific physical signs of chronic fatigue, so a standard physical examination is carried out, with the usual attention to internal organs, lymph glands, heart, lungs and nervous system. Low blood pressure may be a cause of fatigue in its own right, in which case treatment often leads to recovery; but it may also result from the inactivity and deconditioning that occur in CFS. Muscle-wasting may also occur after prolonged inactivity. If pain is a prominent feature, your doctor may check you for fibromyalgia (page 214). It must be said that the physical examination in CFS is usually normal.

LABORATORY INVESTIGATION

There is no diagnostic test for CFS, so the following tests are recommended to exclude other conditions:

- Full blood count (anaemia or other abnormality of blood).
- Erythrocyte sedimentation rate (ESR) or C reactive protein (a marker of inflammation).
- Urea and electrolytes (kidneys and biochemical balance).
- Blood glucose (diabetes or hypoglycaemia).
- Liver function tests.
- Thyroid function tests.
- Creatine kinase (muscle).
- Urine test.

N.B. Other investigations should only be carried out if indicated by individual clinical history or physical examination. The extensive investigation of patients with chronic unexplained fatigue yields no useful information.

Principles of management:

2: Verbalise your beliefs, fears, frustrations and expectations

There are two prevailing illness beliefs that are positively detrimental to patients with chronic fatigue. The first relates to the respective roles of rest and exercise, the second to disease attribution.

It has long been known that prolonged rest is harmful in many situations. In spite of this, rest has been vigorously recommended for patients with CFS. This may be appropriate in the very early stages of acute illness, but prolonged rest leads to physical deconditioning. In particular, the muscles, heart and respiratory system weaken with disuse, and this results in more fatigue. This in turn enforces more rest, leading to more inactivity and further deconditioning. Ironically, graded exercise has been shown by clinical trial to be positively helpful in CFS, but has been actively discouraged by some for fear that it will make things worse. Belief determines behaviour. Thus, patients who believe in the importance of rest and the dangers of exertion, will avoid physical and mental activity, and will unwittingly deepen and prolong their fatigue. On a better day, they may undertake unaccustomed activity and thereafter succumb to post-exertional malaise (made worse because they are so out of condition). Such an experience will reinforce the catastrophic belief that exercise is harmful, and perpetuate the cycle of inactivity, post-exertional malaise, fatigue, and more inactivity. Patients with CFS therefore need to be encouraged towards gradual increments in activity. 'But I was told to listen to my body', you may say; and I reply to that, respectfully, with the empowering suggestion that you can also train your body to 'listen to your mind'.

Disease attribution is important because there is evidence to suggest that those who strongly believe that their illness is purely physical have a greater number of symptoms, and have a poorer prognosis than those who are willing to explore the psychological aspects of their illness. This is not to say that patients are being in any way blamed for their illness, or that their illness is purely psychological. Besides, what if they are right? What if their CFS is very largely physical? Perhaps physical triggers (such as severe infection) do result in a more profound illness than psychological ones (such as bereavement). Nevertheless, this finding does suggest that we should steer clear of the reductionist physical-psychological dichotomy, and embrace a more integrated model — 'the wholistic approach' to treatment.

Patients with CFS express several specific fears. For example, they might be afraid

- of being dismissed. Fatigued patients need an honest expression of acceptance by the doctor that their distress is genuine. Without this, how can they be sure that their fatigue is being taken seriously? Patients also fear dismissal from family, friends and employers, and will value any support their doctor can give them in this regard. The dismissive attitudes of doctors are likely to rub off on those who surround the patient.

- of never getting better. CFS/ME has a formidable reputation for treatment resistance. Some of this has come directly from the medical profession: 'You have ME and there's nothing I can do about it.' The media have also been responsible in as much as they highlight the plight of those who do not improve over time ('I've been house-bound for twenty years with ME') and reinforce dissatisfaction with traditional medical authority. In fact there is good evidence that many patients do eventually recover from CFS, and do get back to work. This is especially true for those who accept and respond to initial treatment, and who adopt healthy illness beliefs and coping styles. The aim here is to maintain a positive attitude and a realistic hope of recovery, although this needs to be balanced against the knowledge that a minority of patients will not do well.

- of passing the illness on to someone else (contagion). Epidemics of CFS are very rare, but still occur. Apart from these, there is no evidence that CFS results in any way from a transmissible agent. However, there is a clinical impression of higher than expected incidences of CFS among first-degree relatives; and twin studies provide further evidence that independent genetic factors may be involved.

- that a diagnosis has been missed. Patients may have difficulty accepting the fact that their distress cannot be explained by physical or laboratory findings, and will express the fear that something has been missed — sometimes to the point of hypochondriasis. The doctor's confidence may be equally undermined. Attention has been drawn to the fact that some conditions, such as occult neoplasm (hidden cancer) or spinal forms of multiple sclerosis, may present with debilitating fatigue and other neuropsychological symptoms long before the underlying disease declares itself. Case reports of mistaken diagnoses do appear from time to time, but these are very rare. The longer you have unexplained fatigue, the less likely it is that something has been missed. This does not alter the fact that extensive investigation without good reason is unhelpful. We should also remember that it is quite possible to develop another illness, entirely unrelated, during the course of CFS. As a precaution, therefore, it is recommended that physical examination and standard laboratory tests be repeated at six to twelve month intervals throughout the course of the illness, particularly when no progress is being made, or if new symptoms should emerge. On the other hand, repeat investigations should be avoided if there are signs of recovery.

- of going mad. Some patients fear they are losing their mind when the doctor tells them they can find nothing wrong. In effect they are saying: How can I be this ill without something to show for it? Be reassured: doctors cannot yet measure fatigue, and that's the only reason they can find no objective evidence of disease. We can find abnormalities in the research setting, but these have not yet been developed into clinical instruments. Thus, we can say that CFS patients, as a group, are not losing their faculties — they have quite specific problems at a molecular level.

- of being forcefully removed into care by the authorities. This applies particularly to affected children and their parents. There have been sad cases of appalling treatment along these lines, where parents are blamed for the 'illness behaviour' of their children. As far as I am aware, this abuse of power is a thing of the past. I trust that by now the professionals involved have developed a greater understanding of the condition.

Finally, CFS is a frustrating condition, and patients express anger towards their doctors for their failure to provide ready answers and cures. But there is no cure! So patients will often do a little 'doctor-shopping' in the hope of finding help. Those who have been dismissed by their own doctors cannot be blamed for moving on; but others may be still looking for the quick fix. We all need to understand that there is a world of difference between cure and functional recovery over time. You will need to come to terms with this frustrating fact. Indeed, perhaps you have not yet come to terms with the diagnosis, let alone what it involves. Are you still struggling with this? It may take you a while to come to a place of acceptance, and you may go through something of a bereavement process on the way. You are grieving the loss of all you formerly enjoyed, and grief will bring you through stages of denial, despair and resignation. The final stage is one of acceptance.

I am not saying here that you have to 'learn to live with it', but I am saying that you need to accept the diagnosis before you can make any real progress. If you remain in denial, you will repeatedly sabotage your own best efforts to recover. Acceptance of the diagnosis, on the other hand, gives you a secure foundation upon which to build an active management plan.

Principles of management:

3. Establish a consistent pattern of sleep, rest and activity

Sleep complaints are common in CFS (and fibromyalgia). These may be attributable to lifestyle or to the condition itself, but they are not solely related to depression or anxiety (even if present). If simple sleep hygiene measures fail to restore a normal sleep–wake schedule with good quality sleep, then we must consider the use of medication. The most useful drugs available to us for this purpose are the antidepressants (see below). Sleeping tablets are not such a good idea, because they can add to daytime fatigue (quite apart from their addictive potential). I know some of you will be unhappy with the notion of antidepressant medication, and I will address these fears shortly. Meanwhile, let us not lose sight of the fact that good sleep is absolutely vital for recovery. So much so that I tell my patients:

- Your first priority is to secure a healthy and consistent sleeping pattern, because
- you cannot expect to feel well until you are sleeping well; and
- having established a pattern, you must strive to maintain it

throughout the entire rehabilitation phase, because
- sleep disruption is *strongly* associated with relapse into fatigue (and fibromyalgia).

We also aim to promote consistency in the areas of rest and activity, and we encourage a gradual and planned increase in activity based on your present level of ability (i.e. the results of your impact assessment). As a general rule, fatigued patients can be encouraged not to abandon the functional activities they have maintained to date, even if they have done so 'in spite of their fatigue'. Thus, those who are still at work should stay at work etc.

Those who are inclined to keep going in spite of their symptoms, and who manage to hold on to some degree of functional activity, will do well in the long run. Conversely, those who are inclined to accommodate their symptoms and who consequently avoid activity for fear of making things worse, will suffer greater disability and prolong their illness. I admit there is potential for conflict and confusion here. On the one hand you are told not to overdo it, and on the other hand you are warned against underdoing it!

The conflict is resolved by the proviso that gradual increments in activity are based on your current level of ability/disability. Thus, whatever the severity of your fatigue, it is always possible to do just a *tiny* bit more. Remember what we said about the 'just noticeable difference' in relation to the perception of effort? It applies here, even in worst case scenarios. The bed-bound, for example, can start with stretching exercises, and then progress to sitting out every day for, say, ten minutes during the first week, increasing to ten minutes twice daily the second week, and so forth. The chair-bound can stand up and take a few steps on the hour, every hour for, say, one minute, increasing to two minutes during the second week, five minutes the third week, and so on. In this manner, even the very debilitated can achieve some degree of functional recovery.

Now, before you protest, consider the alternative. Remain ill and incapacitated? Never! Fight back. You can, ever so gradually, push back the limitations, role constriction and social marginalisation that are intrinsic to states of chronic fatigue. Remember what I said about accepting and responding to initial treatment. Go for it!

Principles of management:

4. Early entry to a graded exercise programme

There are very few interventions which have been shown by clinical trial to be of benefit in CFS, but graded exercise is one of them. For this reason, a formal graded exercise programme should be initiated as soon as possible. This can only be achieved safely and accurately in a gym, or with gym equipment at home. The main work is done on the standard electronic treadmill and the cycle ergometer (bike). Free weights or weight-lifting machines are also used. These allow the doctor and patient to agree on exactly what is being proposed by way of exertion, and they guarantee consistency between one work-out and the next. They also allow us to prescribe very accurate increments in exertion between one week and the next. This reduces the risk of overdoing it.

Each visit to the gym consists of five activities. Start and finish with stretching exercises. The gym instructor will show you how to do these. Stretching should never be painful, so only go as far as you comfortably can, and very gradually increase your flexibility over time. Between the stretching exercises, you walk, cycle and lift weights. The initial speed and duration of the walk, and the duration and resistance of the bike, are educated guesses based on current ability. It is helpful to start off below your current ability. Beware of enthusiastic gym instructors here! They will take one look at you and assume that you are a healthy person trying to get fit — not so. You are a fatigued patient on a prescribed exercise programme trying to get healthy. There is a difference! As you take the very first step on the treadmill, you can say to yourself: 'Right. I have now started on a physical rehabilitation programme. If I give this priority and if it is successful, it will lead me to full recovery.' Any other activity you may wish to do outside of the prescribed programme is for your pleasure only. So, if you fancy going for a walk in the park or a gentle swim, you can go — but you don't have to go. In other words, we make a clear distinction between graded exercise and the other activities of daily life.

The first few weeks of the programme are likely to be boring (because they are not physically challenging). This is quite deliberate. A modest start will help you get used to the social aspects of going out to the gym, and will reassure you that gentle exercise is not harmful. It also provides a safety margin for those who have greater degrees of fatigue and deconditioning, and is less likely to provoke an exercise-induced relapse. As you go through it, remember:

- We appreciate that your (aerobic and anaerobic) exercise tolerance is seriously affected, but the muscles themselves are basically healthy — just deconditioned.
- We also appreciate that patients with CFS have higher perceived exertion scores than the healthy and are therefore being asked to put in a greater (sense of) effort to achieve these goals.
- You can expect some discomfort, fatigue and muscle pain when you start off.
- You may also experience some transient worsening of cognitive impairment, but you will not do yourself any harm by following the prescribed programme.
- You can expect to 'feel' the increments.
- We are aiming for consistency, not heroism.
- Maintain the programme, even on bad days.
- Do not exceed the prescribed exercise, even on good days.
- Graded exercise programmes are used in the management of other well-described medical disorders, including asthma, osteoporosis, cardiac and stroke rehabilitation, diabetes etc.

Once you have embarked on the programme, you can rest assured that you are now actively reclaiming a degree of reliable exertion tolerance; and that this, in turn, will help you reclaim other lost functional ability.

There are only two valid reasons for not going to the gym on a given day. The first is a temperature in excess of 37.5°C, or a resting pulse in excess of 100 beats per minute — both of which could signify current infection. There are also valid reasons for downgrading (readjusting) the exercise programme. If you experience nausea, dizziness or severe pain during exercise, or if you have post-exercise malaise in excess of twenty-four hours, you are probably doing too much. If that is the case, you need a programme with lower exertion demands and more gradual increments. Here is an example of a prescribed exercise

programme, based on a fairly typical patient with CFS who has
maintained mobility and some social function

Name	J. F.	
Age	46 years	
Weight	66 kg	
Minimum weekly expenditure	460 calories	>10 calories per kg body weight/week for health benefits
Maximum weekly expenditure	920 calories	>20 calories/kg body wt/week is of no extra benefit
Frequency of work-outs	3 per week	but could do 5 sessions per week
Minimum daily expenditure	92 calories	
Maximum daily expenditure	184 calories	
Maximal heart rate in health and fitness	174/min.	220-age
Impairment ratio (IR)	1.0	but could be 0.95 or 0.90 depending on previous fitness and present disability
Upper limit heart rate during exercise	130/min.	220-age x 75% x IR (in this case, 1)
Lower limit heart rate during exercise	104/min.	220-age x 60% x IR

Start and finish each session with 10 minutes of stretching
exercises, then . . .

Graded exercise programme — phase I

Week 1.	Walk at	4.0 kph for 10 minutes
	Cycle at	30 watts for 2.5 minutes
	Lift maximum	1 kg for 6 repetitions (1 set)
Week 2.	Walk at	4.5 kph for 10 minutes
	Cycle at	30 watts for 5 minutes
	Lift maximum	1kg for 8 repetitions (1 set)
Week 3.	Walk at	4.5 kph for 15 minutes
	Cycle at	30 watts for 7.5 minutes
	Lift maximum	1 kg for 10 repetitions (1 set)
Week 4.	Walk at	5.0 kph for 15 minutes
	Cycle at	30watts for 10 minutes
	Lift maximum	1 kg for 12 repetitions (1 set)
Week 5.	etc.	

As you can see, the maximum free weight allowed per muscle group is one kilogram — that's the equivalent of one bag of sugar. As an alternative, and if you feel up to it, you could use one plate on the weight-lifting machines instead. Although these are invariably heavier than one kilogram, you will be using several muscle groups to lift it. Use as many machines as you like, but don't exceed the number of repetitions prescribed.

Eventually, the programme will reach the stage where it is no longer possible to walk at a higher speed. This is the time to move up to the second phase of graded exercise: the walk-jog programme. You are now making some real inroads. Here is a sample of what you can expect.

Graded exercise programme — phase II

The time will come when you are walking at your maximum speed. You are now ready to jog. Start each session by cycling at a comfortable pace for ten minutes. Then stretch for ten minutes, and stretch again at the end of the session.

Week 1.	Walk at	6.5 kph x 2.5 minutes, then break into a gentle jog for 30 seconds. Repeat four times, non-stop.
	Weights	3 plates per machine (use all machines in the gym) x 10 repetitions (3 sets)
Week 2.	Walk at	6.5 kph x 2.0 minutes, then break into a gentle jog x 1 minute. Repeat four times, non-stop.
	Weights	3 plates per machine (use all machines in the gym) x 12 repetitions (3 sets)
Week 3.	Walk at	6.5 kph x 1.5 minutes, then break into a gentle jog x 1.5 minutes. Repeat four times, non-stop.
	Weights	3 plates per machine (use all machines in the gym) x 14 repetitions (3 sets)
Week 4.	Walk at	6.5 kph x 1 minute, then break into a gentle jog x 2 minutes. Repeat four times, non-stop.
	Weights	3 plates per machine (use all machines in the gym) x 16 repetitions (3 sets)

Case history

I know this business of graded exercise sounds a little far fetched to the very fatigued. Those who are profoundly disabled may find it impossible to imagine themselves doing any activity, let alone exercise in a gym. I thought, therefore, that you might be encouraged by the real life experience of some of my patients.

Joan is a 32-year-old postgraduate student who came down with chronic fatigue during her final exams, and that was six years ago. She was exhausted, 'absolutely wrecked'. She fought hard to keep going but, in spite of enormous effort, she became more and more debilitated. We tried diets, and they helped for a while; then we tried nutritional supplements and antidepressants of various descriptions; and then many other therapies. The fatigue would not budge. Joan was almost fully house-bound at this stage. She could tell you how many steps there were between her bed and the bathroom, and between the couch and the kitchen. Of course, these steps were measured by *her* gait, so when she said 'seventeen' from bed to bathroom, I knew that meant eight steps for me. Joan's world had contracted with inexorable cruelty from a wide-open space to the confines of her apartment; and even there, she moved only when absolutely necessary.

After several years of fruitless toil, I finally despaired. I didn't like to say it, but I was beginning to think that Joan would never recover. That's when we started a graded exercise programme. We used the principle of the 'just noticeable difference'. Would she really notice the extra effort if she took eighteen steps instead of seventeen? Probably not. Her first exercise was simple: stand every two hours and walk for one minute. Over several months, Joan managed to gradually increase her exercise by very specific and gradual increments. She was careful not to exceed the prescribed work rate on good days, and she forced herself to stick with the programme on bad days. She had several set-backs and we had to reorganise (downgrade) the programme several times, but before long she was managing to take a short daily walk around town. Note this: she had nothing left to give after that! All her available energy went into her exercise programme. She spent the rest of the day either sitting or lying down (but not allowed to sleep). She continued with her programme and did extremely well. I got a letter from her the other day: she's working full-time, she has a full social life and she goes running three times a week, every week!

Joan is what I call a heroine. She put an enormous effort into her rehabilitation. She prioritised her exercise programme, everything else becoming subservient to it. She was determined to win, she never gave up hope, and she never lost sight of her goals. Incidentally, she never became depressed.

I could give many other examples of patients whose lives have been redeemed with the help of graded exercise. For example, I know several patients who are now engaged in competitive rugby, soccer, running, walking and cycling. I even have one patient who completed a marathon, and another who trained for the Olympics! Needless to say, these people were athletic before they became ill. Their involvement in these strenuous pastimes, therefore, is merely an indication of the extent to which they have regained their normal functional activities. Let that be your goal also, to recover everything that you have lost. It is possible.

Principles of management:

5. Treat depression and anxiety, if present

Neuropsychiatric disorders such as depression and anxiety are very common complications of CFS and may affect over half of all patients at some point during their illness. Needless to say, depression and anxiety, if present, should be treated, and treated aggressively if need be. But many patients with CFS are reluctant to accept antidepressant treatment. Some of this stems from the social taboo that still surrounds psychiatric diagnosis and treatment. But in my experience, those who have previously been dismissed as 'just stressed' or 'depressed' are especially reluctant. This is understandable. They reject the dismissive doctor, and rightly so; but they reject the treatment too. Ironically, this may be a case of throwing the baby out with the bath water! I say this because antidepressants can be very helpful in the overall management of CFS, even in the absence of overt depression. Indeed, we could even go further than that and say that all patients with CFS should be offered a trial of appropriate antidepressant medication, particularly if they are failing to make progress with other measures. Many doctors (and their grateful patients) would share this opinion. Antidepressants may help to improve sleep quality, reduce pain and increase energy levels. Besides, antidepressants are used in the management of at least a dozen diverse medical conditions, including migraine, irritable bowel syndrome, neuralgia and other pain disorders, bed-wetting, and even some cases of urticaria (hives).

Patients with fatigue who become depressed can be truthfully told: 'I know depression is not the cause of your fatigue, but you

are depressed now (who wouldn't be?) and we need to treat it.'
Bear in mind:

- There may be a difference between what made you ill (illness-precipitation) and what keeps you ill (illness-perpetuation).
  The fatigue inactivity/deconditioning/fatigue cycle is a clear
  example of this; concomitant mood and sleep disorders should
  be equally clear.
- Research suggests that the appearance of psychiatric disorders
  in patients with CFS can be better understood as a *reaction* to
  the illness, rather than a cause of it; and that the severity of
  psychiatric symptoms is related to the clinical severity of the
  fatigue.
- Neuroendocrine studies provide clear evidence of a
  distinction between CFS and the primary psychiatric
  disorders.

Remember what I said about accepting and responding to initial
treatment. You don't have much control over your response to
medication, but you can decide whether to accept or reject it. My
advice? Go for it! But please be patient. It may take a while to find
the right antidepressant for you.

Principles of management:
6. Treat other medical problems, if present

It makes sense to treat any other concurrent medical condition
that may be present.

- Headache, muscle pain and joint pain are intrinsic
  components of the CFS definition, and may be expected to
  figure prominently in the clinical presentation. These tend to
  become less severe or less troublesome as general progress is
  made. Occasionally they demand specific intervention. No
  formal studies have been published on the subject, but the
  clinical impression is that painkillers, such as non-steroidal
  anti-inflammatory drugs and others, are generally ineffective
  in CFS. They are also ineffective in fibromyalgia, a related
  condition. Antidepressants may be more useful, particularly

when symptoms are associated with sleep disturbance. Once again the choice of drug depends on the global symptom profile of the individual patient.

- Low blood pressure (autonomic dysfunction or neurally mediated hypotension), if prominent and persistent, may benefit from cautious trials of disopyramide or atenolol. Tilt table studies may be considered for patients who are severely affected, particularly if they are prone to regular fainting.
- Recurrent infections are a problem for some and may indicate the need for specific therapy in selected patients (e.g. tonsillectomy).
- Allergic disease is quite common in CFS and may contribute to overall fatigue. Food intolerance has been reported by 13.5 per cent of fatigued patients, and some of these may benefit from formal dietary investigation (the low allergy diet).
- Similarly, irritable bowel syndrome occurs in 50 per cent of patients and can be treated with medication and/or dietary investigation for food intolerance.

Principles of management:

7. Pay attention to psychosocial problems, if present

Although social adversity is not necessarily associated with delayed recovery, it sometimes is. Financial burdens, for example, may be associated with illness severity and perpetuation. Relationship difficulties and unresolved conflicts in the workplace may also need to be addressed. Particular care should be given to psychosocial difficulties which were present prior to and leading up to the illness. They may have contributed to it. It may also be necessary to get help with new difficulties as and when they arise. These could be incidental to the illness or a direct result of it. How does one cope with the loss of friends, income and dignity? And, for that matter, how does one handle the frustrations of any long-term illness? Furthermore, and even without social adversity, the gradual transition from long-term illness to health often involves challenging personal adjustments. Personal counselling may prove very helpful for these aspects of the illness.

Principles of management:

8. Aim for an early return to work, if at all possible

By definition, many patients with CFS will be unable to work, or will be working at reduced capacity. Unemployment directly attributable to CFS is reported in some studies to affect up to 74 per cent of patients, but other reports tell us that 45 per cent still manage to hang on to full-time work, and a further 18 per cent are able for part-time work. However, those who do continue working are likely to

- have more sick leave than their healthy colleagues, with one study suggesting an average loss of sixty-five days per annum among CFS patients.
- report strained relationships at work in relation to disbelief and poor acceptance of the illness.
- say that their work hours have been greatly or moderately reduced by their illness.
- say that the quality and quantity of the work they produce has suffered and is not as good as their previous standard.
- say that the variability of their symptoms affects their work life.
- say that working significantly contributes to their symptoms.
- Say that they get very little sympathy from their employers (compared to patients with other more socially acceptable disabilities).

In spite of the obvious difficulties that CFS patients experience in relation to work, the fact remains that those who do manage to continue working have a better long-term outcome. However, we should interpret this finding with care. Perhaps it's the severity of the illness that predicts a long-term outcome: the worst affected are not able to work, whereas the least affected are. In that case, being able to work simply reflects the severity of the fatigue, rather than the willingness to work. But in any case, the fact remains that working is good for you, even if you are fatigued. You may need to employ a little 'symptom suppression' here in your attempt to persevere. If so, bear in mind what the psychologists told us about the perception of effort: those who can minimise their discomfort (suppress their symptoms) will do better than those who maximise their discomfort (accommodate their symptoms).

For this reason, all patients who have stopped working are encouraged towards an early return to work when the time is right and if at all possible. There is a therapeutic aspect to this. In the first place, you're not sitting around getting more and more frustrated; secondly, you can keep your hand in and your position open; thirdly, you safeguard a minimum income; and finally, you actively fight against the sick role. Having said that, you cannot expect to return to full hours and full productivity overnight. Duties and hours should therefore be restricted to suit individual needs, and gradually increased over time. For example, one such programme might invite the employee to work four hours per day during the first month, increasing by one hour per day per month, until full occupational rehabilitation has been achieved. It must be said that some employers are better at facilitating this than others. Night shifts should be avoided during rehabilitation, as these would quickly interfere with sleep patterns and sabotage your recovery.

Questions are sometimes raised with respect to medical retirement, particularly for those who fail to progress. We are reluctant to agree to this for several reasons. To retire on medical grounds, you have to be able to state that the disorder is permanent, and this we cannot do with CFS. It may take a long time, but the vast majority do eventually recover. More importantly, it is a serious matter for a relatively young person to be categorised as permanently sick. It tends to reinforce the disability. Nevertheless, we must acknowledge the very real difficulties faced by the minority who are simply unable to work. Some insurers are offering these patients medical retirement with annual reviews, and this seems like a reasonable compromise. In these cases the patient is medically retired until such time as they are deemed ready to start a gradual return to gainful employment.

Principles of management:

9. Consider other options for treatment

I said earlier that very few intervention trials have shown benefit in CFS, and that graded exercise was one of them. Well, cognitive behavioural therapy (CBT) is another. CBT differs from counselling in that it is a psychotherapeutic modality which specifically addresses

- Education and explanation of symptoms
- The interaction of illness-perpetuating factors
- Unhelpful illness beliefs and attitudes
- Cognitive reattribution
- Goal-setting and gradual increases in activity
- Lifestyle and problem-solving
- Encouragement towards, and consolidation of achievements.

CBT is an acquired and specific skill for which few therapists have been trained. When properly implemented, some 70 per cent of those who participate in CBT report satisfaction with the process and, more importantly, with the outcome. It helps them to achieve greater goals. I referred in Chapter 2 to the fact that some patients continue to report an increased sense of effort, even after they have made significant progress towards full recovery. CBT would be an excellent way to deal with this problem. Think of it like this: you have been ill for a long time, and you've had to put in a great (sense of) effort to get to where you are now. However, in spite of the fact that you are now doing more and feeling better, you are still used to thinking in terms of the illness. Consequently, the thought of engaging in a given activity evokes subconscious memories of effort, and with them a certain foreboding. CBT will help you change both the perception and the foreboding by helping you to think in terms of your present health and well-being rather than dwell (even subconsciously) on the past illness.

The pragmatic and positive approach to treatment advocated throughout this chapter contains much by way of 'common sense CBT'. But specific CBT, which is only available in a few specialised centres, would seem to be a useful adjunct to treatment. You will need to ask your doctor whether the service is available in your area.

Miscellany

Many other therapies have been advocated for CFS, but very few of these have been subjected to, or withstood, rigorous assessment. Some patients will respond to nutritional supplements, such as the essential fatty acids, together with their supporting (transport) nutrients, vitamin C, coenzyme Q10 and carnitine. Others may benefit from magnesium injections, but results are mixed. Any patient who has symptoms that could be related to diet should consider dietary investigation for food intolerance, or an empirical trial of the gut fermentation regime. Claims have also been made for many other interventions far too numerous to go through in detail. For example, eNADH, estrogens, light therapy and selegiline have all been said to help some patients, but not others.

Principles of management:

10. Maintain a positive attitude and a realistic hope for recovery

The vast majority of CFS patients can expect to regain a significant quality of life. Some 25 per cent or more will get to the stage where they consider themselves fully and absolutely recovered — as if they were never ill in the first place. Four out of five patients can expect to get back to gainful employment. One in five may experience slower progress and a greater struggle, but even these will improve over time. Very few remain ill for years. What can you do to improve your chances of a successful outcome? Accept and respond to initial treatment.

Section 5

Overcoming Fatigue

Chapter 26 In Pursuit of Relief

26   In Pursuit of Relief

Having read through the previous chapters, you may be left wondering where to start in your pursuit of relief. On the other hand, you may have found 'your' chapter — the one that best describes your condition and suggests the most likely diagnosis. In any case, this short chapter hopes to provide you with a simple step-by-step guide through the various measures you can take to shake off your fatigue, improve your energy levels and secure a better quality of life. These are presented under two headings, namely, lifestyle issues and medical concerns.

Lifestyle issues

Adopt the following lifestyle changes for a period of six consecutive weeks and enjoy the difference.

1. Cut out caffeine, smoking and alcohol

Your first step, whatever your combination of symptoms, is to exclude all caffeine from your diet. This includes the obvious tea and coffee, as well as the less obvious caffeine-loaded soft drinks and chocolate. This drug can interfere directly with sleep patterns, mood, energy levels and other bodily functions. Remember to wean yourself off tea and coffee slowly, gradually reducing your intake over a two week period. This will help reduce the withdrawal symptoms. If you cannot imagine life without these drinks, you are indeed an addict! Such addiction is a clear indication that you do need to give up the habit, at least for a while. It would be better initially not to drink decaffeinated substitutes, as these may also affect health. You would also be well advised to give up smoking and reduce your alcohol consumption significantly, if not altogether, as these may cause fatigue in susceptible persons.

2. Get enough sleep

At the risk of patronising again, the next step is to examine your sleep pattern, and to distinguish between the feelings of excessive daytime sleepiness and fatigue. If you are not waking up every morning feeling refreshed, you must ask yourself the most basic of questions: are you getting enough sleep? Determine your sleep requirement, as outlined on pages 78-9, and make sure you get your full quota for these six weeks. If you are starting from a point of sleep debt, try going to bed early (8 or 9 p.m.) every night for a week. During this time, rise early (8 a.m.) and take a walk just before or after breakfast. If you suspect that you have a primary sleep disorder, ask your doctor to confirm, and consider referral to a sleep disorder specialist.

3. Take regular exercise

The healthy find exercise invigorating. Spending energy increases energy! The fatigued will also benefit from exercise, so long as the exertion is reasonable and with gradual increments. Start with daily walks and gradually increase the distance covered each week. If necessary, start a formal graded exercise programme. If you like, you can partake in more strenuous activity (sports), particularly if you are used to doing so, and if you are not too severely affected. You will need to be careful with this: sporty people frequently underestimate their degree of fatigue. Avoid any activity which leaves you feeling totally drained, but do build up your exertion tolerance slowly.

4. Eat a healthy diet

By a healthy diet, I mean one which provides you with all the essential nutrients. Eat plenty of fruit and vegetables, as well as meat, fish, milk, cheese, nuts, cereals, and complex carbohydrates such as potato and rice. You would do well to implement the food pyramid on page 105. Eat regular nutritious meals, and do not go for long periods without food. A course of nutritional supplementation (a tonic) could also be considered, but get advice on this.

If you have symptoms of hypoglycaemia, exclude all highly refined carbohydrates such as sweets, biscuits, cake and ice cream etc. Eat something every one or two hours, as detailed in Chapter 17.

5. Identify the stress, and deal with it

Obviously, it is important to be aware of the varied pressures you are under at the moment, whether they be sleepless young children, financial hardship, employment worries, relationship problems or personal dissatisfaction. It is all too easy to drift in times of stress. We struggle on and on, hoping it will just go away, but it won't. It is far better to take a positive approach. Take time out, and examine those things that are going on inside you at a deeper level. You may be surprised at how much benefit can be derived from an honest appraisal of real issues. To this end, a professional counsellor will be invaluable. Remember that your first visit is very much a two-way interview. You assess the counsellor just as much as s/he assesses you. You will be looking for someone you can trust and feel comfortable with; they will be trying to find out what's going on, and whether they feel they can help you. If you are not happy with the first counsellor you meet, try another — shop around. Once you have found a suitable person, s/he will probably offer you a 'contract' of, say, six weekly visits. By the end of this time, you will both be in a position to decide on the relative benefits of continuing in therapy. The more profound depressions may require antidepressant medication, but stay away from the long-term use of tranquillisers if possible.

6. Relax and get some space

Relaxation exercises can only do you good. Follow the breathing exercise procedure in Chapter 6. This is not only relaxing in itself, but it will help to correct the chemical imbalances of hyperventilation. The procedure must be followed for twenty minutes twice a day, every day, for the best results. It is also appropriate to arrange space for yourself in which you can pursue an enjoyable pastime or hobby.

Medical issues

If your fatigue is profound and/or accompanied by other symptoms, you may have to do more than simply change your lifestyle.

7. Investigate the possibility of food intolerance

Hidden food reactions may interfere directly with sleep, mood and energy levels. You may therefore decide to defer counselling and/or further medical investigation until after you have tried a low allergy diet. Follow the diet outlined in Chapter 15 for a period of seven to ten days. If you have no relief from this and you still think that food is a problem, try eating lamb and pears for seven days. If your symptoms remain, they are not caused by food! Please do not restrict your diet in the long term unless there is indisputable evidence of benefit from doing so, and get expert dietary advice to ensure adequate nutrition.

8. Consider a gut fermentation control regime

If you have no immediate and substantial relief from your symptoms on the low allergy diet, and if you have the symptoms of gut fermentation, move straight on to the stage 1 gut fermentation control diet, as given in Chapter 18. You will need a doctor's help if you are going to do this properly. Nystatin powder is a prescription-only medicine, and you will need expert advice on nutritional supplements. Some authorities insist that the diet be adhered to for six months before you decide that it has failed you. I personally recommend that you do not go beyond two months unless there is obvious benefit from it.

9. Chemical-free holidays

If you have any hint of chemical sensitivity, you should consider arranging a chemical-free holiday in the early days of the low allergy and gut fermentation control diets. If your symptoms improve when you are away from chemicals, and return again when you are subsequently exposed, create a chemical-free environment in your home. If necessary, remove fuel-burning boilers to an outhouse. Once again, be careful not to incur great expense until you are sure that it's worth it.

10. Medical help

If your fatigue persists in spite of all these measures, you must now consult a doctor — preferably one with a particular interest in fatigue states. What you need, above all else, is to be given unhurried time by a sympathetic physician, who will not only listen to your story, but believe it as well! The usual ten minute (if you're lucky) consultation in the middle of a busy surgery is woefully inadequate as far as fatigue is concerned. It may take you half an hour or longer to go through the details of your symptoms. At this stage, a physical examination and a few basic blood tests are mandatory. If these draw a blank, and if your symptoms warrant it, you may need to see a hospital specialist and undergo further investigation. If all these results are normal — as they often are — do not be disappointed. It is a good thing that no nasty disease has been found. You will probably be asked to see a psychiatrist now! Go. Let them ask you all the questions they want, and be honest with your answers. You have nothing to hide. But before you go, ask your specialist if you fulfil the diagnostic criteria for CFS, and enquire about parasites.

If you do have CFS or a related disorder, ask to see a doctor with a specialist interest in these conditions. And above all, remember that most people will recover fully, given time, support and suitable medical advice.

Appendix 1.
An Effective
Treatment for Allergy

I would like to pay homage to Dr Len McEwen, the pioneer who developed a very specific and effective treatment for allergy, namely, enzyme potentiated desensitisation, or EPD for short.

The story of EPD goes back to 1959, and to the London office of an ear, nose and throat surgeon named Popper. He was interested in nasal polyps, those grape-like structures that can block a nose. He knew that polyps consisted mainly of a gooey substance called hyaluronic acid, and he figured that if he could dissolve the acid, the polyp would shrink and the patient could avoid surgery. Nice thought! He injected his patients' nasal polyps with an enzyme (hyaluronidase) which he hoped would break down the acid. When they returned for a progress report, they volunteered that their polyps were still there, *but some of them had stopped sneezing*. In other words, the injection had desensitised them. They no longer had allergic rhinitis. Popper then tried to repeat his experiment with another batch of hyaluronidase and another batch of patients. However, this time he failed to desensitise. Sadly, his work was cut short by an untimely death. That would have been the end of the story if it were not for the ingenuity and persistence of Dr Len McEwen. He knew from Popper's work that hyaluronidase was not the important ingredient, and he realised that the first batch must have been contaminated with some other active ingredient. He went back to the first batch and found six contaminants. By trial and error he found the gem, an enzyme called beta-glucuronidase. He successfully desensitised both animals and man to various allergens, and he published his findings in the medical literature. He has devoted his working life to the further development of this treatment.

What is EPD?

EPD is a desensitisation treatment for allergy and intolerance. It consists of a mixture of beta-glucuronidase and allergens. The enzyme is already present in our bodies and has powerful immune system effects. The allergen mixtures include commonly eaten foods, airborne allergens, chemicals, and a few 'odds and ends'. Each patient will receive the allergen mixture best suited to his/her needs.

How does it work?

A very small amount (0.05 ml) of EPD solution is injected between two layers of skin. The enzyme stimulates special cells in the skin called antigen-presenting cells (APCs). These 'wake up' to find themselves bathed in the allergen mixture. They lay hold of the allergens and migrate to the immune system 'headquarters'. Their job in life is to present allergen and ask for judgment: 'Do we ignore this allergen or do we mount an immune response against it?' Because the APCs are primed with beta-glucuronidase, the immune system responds favourably to the allergen, realises there is no threat to health, and organises a truce. A new population of cells is then called forth with instructions not to react in the presence of these allergens. These cells are called T suppressor cells. They have the power of a military police force, and they suppress other components of the immune system which would otherwise react to the allergen. T suppressor cells suppress allergic reactions.

What is it used for?

EPD has been used successfully in the treatment of hay fever, asthma, perennial rhinitis, nasal polyps, urticaria and angioedema, as well as food-induced hyperactivity, migraine, irritable bowel syndrome, Crohn's disease, ulcerative colitis, eczema and arthritis. It has also helped some patients with chronic fatigue syndrome. EPD has not yet been developed for the treatment of contact allergic dermatitis, drug allergy or insect sting allergy.

Is it safe?

The amount of allergen administered with each dose of EPD is never greater than the dose you would receive with a diagnostic skin prick test. For this reason, EPD is a very safe treatment. Patients with a history of life-threatening allergic reactions are offered an even greater degree of safety — an epidermal scrape. This consists of superficially scraping the skin with the edge of a blunted scalpel. A sterile plastic 'cup' is then taped over the scrape and filled with EPD treatment. The solution is allowed to percolate through the skin for twenty-four hours and the cup is then removed. Some fluid may still be present and a jelly-like substance may cover the scrape. This will dry within thirty minutes, and the scrape will heal normally over the next ten days or so. There have been no serious side effects from EPD since its inception some thirty years ago.

Are there any side effects?

It is quite normal for the injection site to swell immediately after injection. This will quickly subside. A delayed swelling may also occur after three to six hours and may persist for three days, but it should begin to subside by the fourth day. Very rarely, the whole forearm may swell. These are not serious reactions and they respond to antihistamine tablets. Other side effects include a transient worsening of the allergies being treated, such as sneezing, runny nose, urticaria etc. These will usually disappear within a few days, but may persist in some cases for a few weeks and, very rarely, for a few months. Patients undergoing a course of EPD are given detailed instructions. This will increase their chance of success and keep side effects to a minimum.

Is it effective?

EPD has been shown by clinical trial to be effective in up to 80 per cent of patients. In other words, four out of five patients, whose allergies have been properly identified, will enjoy some benefit from treatment.

How long will it be before improvement?

It takes about twenty-one days for the newly stimulated T-cells to mature. There will usually be no appreciable difference in your allergic symptoms until this time has elapsed. The response to the first dose of EPD is variable — most patients will experience some benefit, but some may not, and some may even feel worse. Patients with eczema, hyperactivity and chronic fatigue syndrome are most likely to report a definite, albeit transient, worsening of symptoms after their first dose of EPD. Subsequent doses do not have a negative effect.

How many injections will I need?

Simple allergies such as house dust mite will respond to two or three injections. Significant relief from hay fever may be obtained by just one or two injections given well before the hay fever season starts. Other conditions may require four injections (or more) before any real improvement is noticed. Injections are given at eight to twelve week intervals until a good response is obtained. Then, depending on the response, further injections are given at ever increasing intervals. Once their symptoms are well controlled, most patients find that they can stop injections for very long periods. Relapses may occur after five or six years, but these respond to booster doses.

EPD, not to be confused with blocking desensitisation

Blocking desensitisation is a technique which involves the injection of allergen in incremental doses. The first injection is small, the second is a little stronger etc. This system of desensitisation floods the immune system with allergen and provokes the production of a 'blocking antibody'. This is an immuno-globulin which saturates the mast cells and basophils, and in so doing prevents their degranulation by IgE. The system was developed in the late nineteenth century. It works well and is still used today throughout continental Europe and North America. However, it has caused a number of deaths from anaphylaxis. For this very good reason, blocking desensitisation is not used at all in Ireland, and only in highly specialised centres in the United Kingdom. The technique is limited to specific allergens, such as grass pollen, insect venom and house dust mite. EPD uses much smaller doses than blocking desensitisation, and for this reason is a much safer technique. It also has a wider scope in that it can be used for many allergens simultaneously.

Appendix 2.
Useful Addresses

Action Against Allergy
P.O. Box 278
Twickenham
Middlesex TW1 4QQ

Anaphylaxis Campaign (Ireland)
P.O. Box 4373
Dublin 18
Tel: 01 2952791

Anaphylaxis Campaign (UK)
P.O. Box 149
Fleet
Hants GU13 9XU
Tel: 01252 318723

Biolab Medical Unit
The Stone House
Weymouth Street
London W1N 3FF
Tel: 0207 6365959

British Association for Counselling
1 Regent Place
Rugby
Warwickshire CV21 2PJ

British Society for Allergy, Environmental and Nutritional Medicine
P.O. Box 28
Totton
Southampton SO40 2ZA
Tel: 02380 812124

Irish ME Trust
18 Upper Fitzwilliam Street
Dublin 2
Tel: 01 6761413

Irish ME Support Group
Tel: 01 2350965

ME Association (UK)
Stanhope House
High Street
Stanford-le-Hope
Essex SS17 0AH
Tel: 01375 642466

Pesticide Exposure Group of Sufferers
3 Lloyd's House
Regent Terrace
Cambridge CB2 1AA
Tel: 01223 64707

Psychological Society of Ireland
13 Adelaide Road
Dublin 2
Tel: 01 4783916

Bibliography

Candidiasis 2nd Edition
Gerald P. Bodey
Raven Press, New York.
ISBN 0 88167 954 2

Chemical Exposures, Low Levels High Stakes, 2nd Edition
Nicholas Ashford and Claudia Miller
Van Nostrand Reinhold, 115 Fifth Avenue, New York, NY 10003.
ISBN 0 442 02524 6

Chronic Fatigue: your complete exercise guide
Neil F. Gordon
Human Kinetics Publishers.

Chronic Fatigue and its Syndromes
Simon Wessely, Matthew Hotopf, Michael Sharpe
Oxford University Press.
ISBN 0 19 262181 5

Clinical Management of Chronic Fatigue Syndrome
Nancy Klimas, Roberto Patarca, Eds
The Haworth Medical Press, New York.
ISBN 1 56024 792 4

Coping with Chronic Fatigue
Trudie Chalder
Sheldon Press, London.
ISBN 0 85969 685 5

Bibliography

Could it be an Allergy?
Dr Joe Fitzgibbon
Newleaf.
ISBN 0 7171 2682 X

Diagnostic and Statistical Manual of Mental Disorders IV
America Psychiatric Association
Washington, DC.
ISBN 0 89042 062 9

Environmental Medicine in Clinical Practice
Anthony H., Birtwistle S., Eaton K., Maberly J.
BSAENM Publications, P.O. Box 28, Totton, Southampton SO40 2ZA.
ISBN 0 9523397 2 2

Food Allergy and Intolerance
Jonathan Brostoff and Stephen J. Challacombe
Balliere Tindall, London.
ISBN 0 7020 1156 8

Framing Disease, Studies in Cultural History
Charles E. Rosenberg and Janet Golden, Eds
Rutgers University Press, New Brunswick, New Jersey.
ISBN 0 8135 1756 7

Manual of Nutrition 10th Edition
Ministry of Agriculture, Fisheries and Food
The Stationery Office, London.
ISBN 0 11 242991 2

Nutritional Medicine
Dr Stephen Davies and Dr Alan Stewart
Pan Books.
ISBN 0 330 28833 4

Perceived Exertion
Bruce J. Noble and Robert J. Robertson
Human Kinetics, P.O. Box IW14, Leeds LS16 6TR, UK.
ISBN 0 88011 508 4

Bibliography

Post-Viral Fatigue Syndrome
Rachel Jenkins and James Mowbray, Eds
John Wiley & Sons, Chichester.
ISBN 0 471 92846 1

Postviral Fatigue Syndrome
Behan P.O., Goldberg D.P., Mowbray J.F., Eds
British Medical Bulletin, Vol. 47, Number 4, Oct. 1991
Churchill Livingston.
ISBN 0 443 044902

Present Knowledge in Nutrition 7th Edition
Ziegler E.E., Filer L.J., Eds
ILSI Press, Washington, DC.
ISBN 0 944398 72 3

Principles and Practice of Sleep Medicine 3rd Edition
Kryger M.H., Roth T., Dement W.C., Eds
W.B. Saunders Co.
ISBN 0 7216 7670 7

Stress, the Immune System and Psychiatry
Brian E. Leonard, Klara Miller, Eds
Wiley & Sons, Chichester.
ISBN 0 471 95258 3

Index